Pushing the Boundaries

Memoirs of a Travelled Doctor

Penelope Key

*Jenny*
*with my love*
*Penel (1 Nov. 09)*

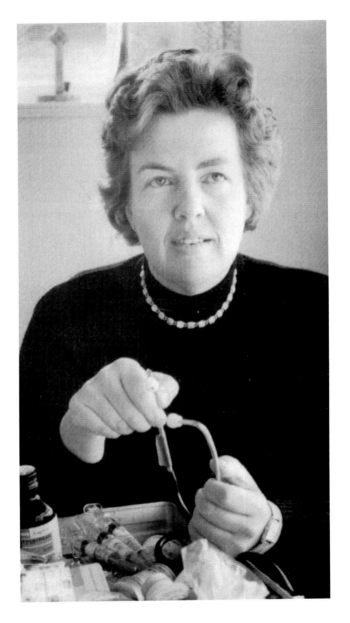

*Myself as a young doctor*

Produced in association with
Christine Holmes

*Bound Biographies*

Heyford Park House
Bicester
OX25 5HD
www.boundbiographies.com

ISBN: 978-1-905178-35-3

Printed in Great Britain by the
MPG Books Group, Bodmin and King's Lynn

## Dedication

To Jane, Sophy and Helen,
who are all professional women in their fields of
service. I am confident they will continue in the
tradition of their ancestors and their
family of women who served their communities
and country so well.

In memory of Drs Kim Nguon and Bun Thol
who lost their lives in Cambodia while serving
their people

## Acknowledgements

To my brother, John –
for his foreword and helpful comments

To my sister, Kem Kanyaket, 'Kan' –
for her story and encouragement

To my cousins, Ann and Haydn –
for their encouragement and thorough reading of
the manuscript

And to Christine Holmes–
for her support and advice

*This has been a big story to tell, much of it from memory.*
*Any inaccuracies are solely my responsibility.*

# FOREWORD

Family chronicles are rare, but very precious. When my mother Joan published *Stover – The Story of a School* in 1982, she birthed a resource that has informed and enlightened three generations of people, whose lives have been impacted by Stover. Now, to my delight, my sister Pene has given us *Pushing the Boundaries – Memoirs of a Travelled Doctor*, through which she invites us to share her journey of forty-five years and some of her amazing experiences in different parts of the world. It is a powerful, absorbing and colourful story.

It has been my privilege to watch Dr Pene at work in places like Dogura, a remote mission station in Papua New Guinea; and Bhubaneswar in Orissa, one of India's poorest states; and Phnom Penh, Cambodia's capital as it recovered from the trauma of the Pol Pot era. She was consistently authoritative, passionate and dogged. She knows her stuff, she cares deeply for the people she is serving and she sees the task through to its completion. Whatever the problems, the boundaries get pushed out. Sustained by her Christian faith, she is fearful of nobody, least of all intransigent males!

I believe there are hundreds of thousands of people on our planet who owe their quality of life, even life itself, to the health interventions and preventive systems that Pene has helped governments and other agencies put in place in the two-thirds world. Not that she has finished. As the last chapter makes clear, she is planning the next ten years, with malaria control, stroke research and more international projects in her sights.

*Pushing the Boundaries* is a wonderful chronicle of past adventures and achievements, but its primary purpose is about the future and the potential of the rising generations. Pene has dedicated her book to her three nieces, Jane, Sophy and Helen, who are all making a significant difference in their worlds of child and family protection, veterinary medicine and the education of teenagers. She is challenging Imogen, Phoebe, Libby, Holly, Olivia, Ella, Laura, Clare and others yet unborn to rise up and push out the boundaries as they take their place as future leaders. Not to mention the many male Keys as well! There is a bright future for family chronicles.


John Key
Sydney, Australia
April 2009

# Contents

# Chapter 1: Family background and my early years

This book is intended for my much-loved nephews and nieces and their children; and in recognition of my family heritage, I intend to write enough to give a family context, before writing my own personal story.

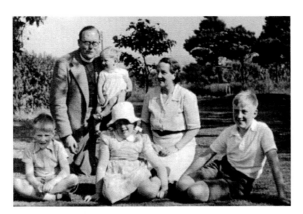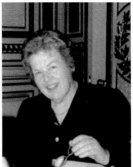

*The family about 1947 and a later photo of me at a conference dinner*

Some people say that, when a group of our family gathers, there is a likeness to be seen – particularly among the women. In the same way, I believe there are threads of temperament and other likenesses that can be traced. I will not go back further than my parents' parents, as I did not know any of my great-grandparents, but this much will give my nephews and nieces – and 'greats' – quite a significant line to follow.

My father's father was Frederick John Key who was a rector all his adult life. He married Dorothy Head, from a relatively wealthy family in Hexham, Northumberland. Frederick and Dorothy had seven or eight children, of whom two died in infancy, and the one who would have become my Uncle Basil died at the age of six, of diphtheria. In fact, the whole family except my father suffered heart disease, a legacy of rheumatic illness in their childhood – a consequence of being brought up in poverty and living in the cold, damp vicarages of the Potteries area of Staffordshire where my grandfather spent most years of his working life. The two surviving daughters were my Aunt Joyce, who became a teacher, and Aunt Winifred, always known to us in the family as 'Gui', after the country of Guiana, where she worked as a teacher for the government, as I tell later. The two brothers were my Uncle Oswald (always called 'OJ'), a teacher, and Uncle Brian who was a civil servant in the Ministry of Food.

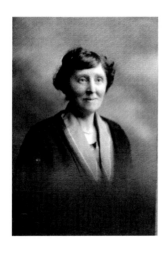

*Granny Key, née Dorothy Head (Father's mother)*

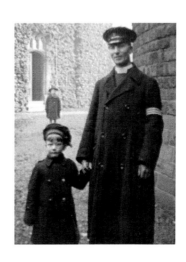

*Grandfather Frederick Key with Basil*

My grandfather was in poor health (probably a bad chest) and needed to get away from Staffordshire, so came south to Aylesbeare near Exeter in Devon, where he was rector for just one year. Then he died and was buried in a family grave at Aylesbeare, and my father, who was recently ordained, became rector in his place. After a while, Father was appointed to the church at Highweek, near Newton Abbot. It was while he was there that, in his early thirties, he fell for the headmistress of Stover School, where he was chaplain. More of that later... My father was the only one of his family who married, and I remember many visits from the single aunts and uncles when I was young.

I need to mention here that my mother's relationship with her mother-in-law was not the best. Granny Key was chronically ill with rheumatoid arthritis and was very disabled by it. In those days, the only treatment was 'gold injections' which made little difference and were painful. I remember what a terrible struggle it was for Granny to walk at all, and she had no one to look after her as both her daughters were away working. Granny thought the world of my dad – understandably. I think my mother's problem was that Granny resented their marriage, as it broke up her new home. She had just moved to Highweek Rectory to be with her son, my father, when he got married and brought in his new, young wife, my mother. Granny had to find somewhere else to live and she never did have another home of her own, existing in boarding houses until her death.

On my mother's side, my grandfather was Arthur Thomas Dence (the name is from a French Huguenot family – earlier spelt Dens). Arthur became a successful businessman, whose company produced Brands Essence, and he married Ethel Mary Searle in London, and it is from this line that the family likeness, the Dence look, is traced. He was obviously a man of great principle and later was ordained a minister. He died quite young (in his sixties) in Torquay, having moved to make his home in Devon some years before. There is a story to tell about him: Grandfather and his large family lived in *Court Grange*, a large house in Abbotskerswell near Newton Abbot, until the day when he heard of a blind babies' home in Kent being destroyed by fire. This news must have been on the wireless and it touched him, so that he announced to the family gathered for breakfast the next morning, that he had given the house away... The house remained a home for blind children for many years but later was given to the Deaf Association.

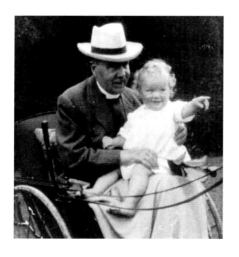

*Grandfather Dence –
in a bath chair with
granddaughter Helen
Mary*

But back to my grandparents Arthur and Ethel. My Granny Dence was a character of substantial proportions. She always wore long dresses and some of us children even wondered if she had legs. She and Grandfather had seven daughters and two sons. The eldest, my Uncle Frank, married and had two children, but I rarely met them. The other brother, my Uncle Arthur, ran away to Australia, and it was he whom my Aunt Phyllis took me to meet after her retirement – and that lead to my life overseas. The girls were all strong-minded and well educated, which was unusual for girls before the First World War.

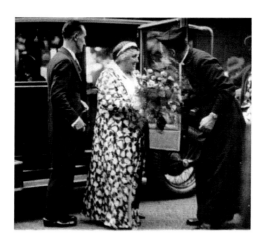

*Granny Dence – at my parents' wedding, 1935*

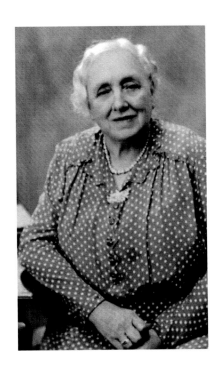

*Granny Dence:*
*the family 'look'*

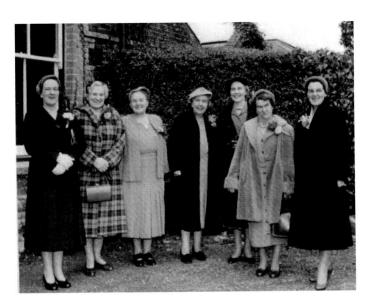

*The Dence sisters, 1955.  L-R: Joan, Irene, Doris, Ruth, Phyl, Pearl*
*and Audrey*

Aunt Doris was the first, and she went off to become a nurse. She married a young man who worked for the British and Foreign Bible Society in Palestine. During the first year of married life, they lived in Beirut, where Doris at once put her nursing to excellent use. Later she and her husband went to Argentina. They had four children, and I have grown close to Peggy, who went to Pakistan and the Sudan, and worked there with her husband, something which has given us a lot in common.

\*\*\*

Aunt Ruth married a farmer in Dorset and I was very fond of her. We would sometimes go and stay with them, and I remember the food on the farm, especially the butter and cream, as being particularly good – something that was significant to those of us who were used to wartime shortages.

\*\*\*

Then there was Aunt Rene who ran a nursing home at Weymouth for a while. She had a daughter Susan, the same age as me.

\*\*\*

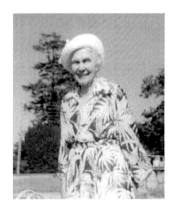

*Aunt Phyllis*
*at Stover*

The next was Aunt Phyllis, 'Aunt Do', who was closest to Mother and who had a great influence on my life. In fact, she influenced all of us with her love of music and her devotion to it, making sure her nephews and nieces learned something of it. She was educated at Cheltenham Ladies' College and went on to study and gain a degree from the Royal College of Music. She never married, but often stayed and even came on holiday with us. When my mother needed to find a successor at Stover, Aunt Phyllis stepped in and she was headmistress there for twenty-five years.

\*\*\*

16

Then came my mother Agnes Joan (or 'Jo'), who was also educated (although briefly) at Cheltenham Ladies' College. She was not scholastic but studied at Bible college in Bristol with the intention of becoming a missionary. When she went home to Torquay as a young woman of about twenty, my grandfather, who disliked idleness and insisted that any of his family living at home should find useful things to do, suggested she start a school for the young children of her friends. Mother was not trained to teach, but she obviously had a strong faith and a practical mind, as seen very clearly in her successfully founding a school which began in rented accommodation at *The Chestnuts*, in Newton Abbot, but before long had grown significantly. The tale is told in my mother's book, *Stover – The Story of a School*, where there is also an account of the 'red-haired rector of Highweek' falling in love with her. I have not told a lot of their history together, but theirs was a very happy marriage that lasted nearly fifty years.

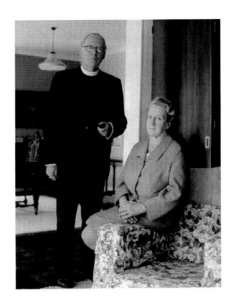

*Portrait of my parents*

***

Aunt Audrey was one of the very early women doctors, so had the same interest in medicine as is seen in others of the family. She specialised in maternal and child health and worked in the service dedicated to that. My mother used to say she was 'not a proper doctor as she did not see patients'!

17

Aunt Audrey married a man who became a headmaster and they lived in Tavistock, Stockport and finally Hampton, and had four children. I really grew up with these four – and Ann, who was the same age as me, was almost a sister.

***

The last in my grandparents' family was Aunt Pearl, who had an illness when she was born and became spastic and seriously physically handicapped. She was a woman of great spirit and fun. She loved a good laugh and lived to a fine old age, and was a good friend to my brothers and me.

***

## And now, for my own story …

Over the last few years, as I have struggled to come to terms with a stroke and chronic ill health, I have wondered if I spent my lifetime right – if indeed I have made a difference to the countries and people I have tried to serve. What has been the value of my service to the people in those countries where I have worked – and even at home? This account of my life's work is an attempt to evaluate and justify myself to myself, and also to tell the next generation of my family (and generations to come) just what Auntie Pene spent her time doing on her travels overseas – especially in remote and warring countries. There will be many stories passed around, but this is what actually happened in my life.

When I was born, in Highweek Rectory, Newton Abbot, my parents intended to call me Elizabeth Joan Key. My mother told me that the day before my baptism, her sister Phyllis Elizabeth (after whom I was being named), contacted her and my father, saying she had heard the name Penelope, which she thought was lovely. There were too many Elizabeths, and please would they change my name at baptism – to Penelope Joan? They instantly agreed and I was baptised at three months, 'Penelope Joan'. My father didn't want me called 'Penny' – he decided that 'Pene' was original and insisted that I always wrote my name 'Pene' – rather a trial for me sometimes. In the family I am usually just 'Pen'.

My brother John was already eighteen months old and my second brother Timothy followed me after seventeen months. My third brother Robert came along seven years later – a post-war baby.

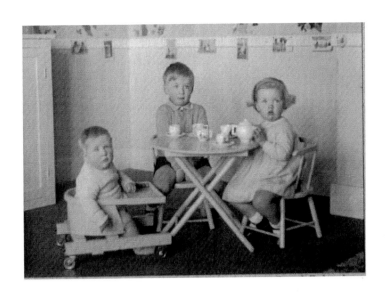

*With brothers John and Timothy, c 1941*

We were a happy rectory family, without much money, but surrounded by love. Like my father, my mother was a committed Christian, and she taught us to sing hymns and read us Bible stories on Sundays. My father was a mild, humble man – especially devoted to me, I think.

He called me Pen or 'Tumps' – short for Stumpy, from the way I walked. He was a rare letter-writer, and in his letters he always addressed me as VPD or even VVPPD – a joke between us, standing for Very Precious Daughter.

My father never got angry with the boys or me: my mother was our disciplinarian. Family legend has it that the only time Father ever raised his hand to any of us was to John, aged three years, when he deliberately rode his tricycle over me – a well-upholstered baby, rolling on the grass lawn at Stover. I think it would have been pretty impossible – and whatever he did, it had no ill-effects that I know of. He got a good spanking from my father.

Born in 1938, I have war memories. We moved to Devonport, Plymouth, in 1940 and were immediately caught up in the heavy raids on the docks. I remember, though I was only three or four, going to bed in our cellars and even hearing the sound of the guns – which scared me. I remember incendiary bombs and forming human chains with buckets of water to put out the fires.

19

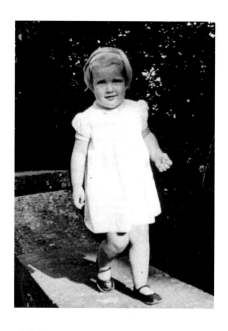

*A little girl, VPD,*
*with a big purpose*

We children and our nanny (Vi) were evacuated from Plymouth to friends in the country at Bovey Tracey in 1941 – and then began a series of moves from friend to friend through the war years. Our rectory in Devonport had three direct hits soon after we left. My mother, who came with us to the country, used to watch the red skies to the west with great fear, wondering what was happening to my father. He was an ARP warden and spent many nights on the rooftops of Devonport putting out incendiary fires. He used to tell us how one night he was at home, having a smoke and taking a stroll before bed with his brother OJ who was visiting, when the sirens went and he looked up to the planes overhead – dropping bombs.

He was fixated by one bomb hurtling down and knew it was coming for him. He dived for the cellar, and the impact of the bomb as it hit our house blew him down the steps into the cellar, from where he and OJ were rescued unhurt next day. Our house took three hits that night. To this day we have old tables with holes caused by shrapnel. My mother, visiting next day, said she opened the glass cupboard, containing mostly precious glass wedding presents, expecting the worst, only to find every glass intact. Our cut glass became very precious after that.

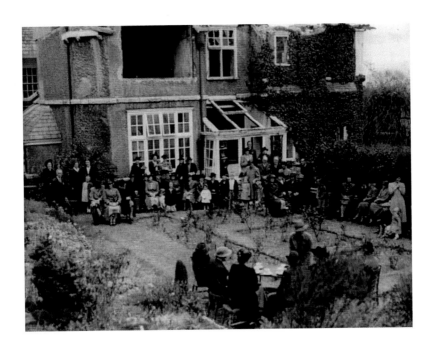

*Our bombed rectory, 1940*
*Our family is in the corner by the conservatory*

Over the next months, the three of us were passed around friends locally. Staying in Bovey Tracey, I started school with John, at Stover. We used to walk every morning with Vi in attendance, down the steep slope of Hind Street to the railway station (now closed). From there we steamed along the short distance to Teigngrace station, where we got off and were 'bussed' up the drive to Stover House. A little later, Tim was sent with us and John and I were given charge of him, though he was a naughty yet enterprising child.

Stover at that time was the site of a large American military camp, swarming with soldiers and weapons. We had to show special passes to the soldiers before we were allowed to pass up the drive. One fateful day, Tim did not have his and, at all of three years old, he was taken off the bus as if he were an alien. We were terrified of course, but he soon turned up at the police station.

We moved back to Devonport in 1944, when the worst was over for Plymouth. Our new house had an amazing view over Plymouth Sound and we were mesmerised watching the warships sailing in and out. We benefited from ship parties – given for the deprived children of Plymouth – where we were introduced to treats such as chocolate and ice cream. We did not like the bananas. I am supposed to have eaten thirteen ice creams myself at one party!!

John and I were sent to a dame school in Devonport. The elderly Miss Collins took about six children and we were drilled in maths and spelling. This grounding has stood us both well all our lives.

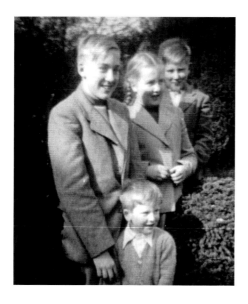

*With my brothers*
*about 1948*

In 1947, after my brother Robert was born, my father was called to be a bishop in the church and we all moved to Salisbury for the next ten years. I had a very happy childhood there, totally involved in the life and community of the great Cathedral and its Close. It was here that I accepted and stepped forward in my Christian faith, which has remained strong all my life. We all went to day schools in Salisbury (I to Godolphin School), though it was always understood that the boys would go away to boarding school at thirteen. That was when I began to rebel. Why the boys and not me? Unfair! Ever since then I have promoted gender equality at home and at work. I was disgusted when my father declared that 'ladies first' all the time was a bit hard in a family with three boys and one girl. He introduced a rule in our house that on Sundays it was 'boys first'. At Sunday lunch, my brothers were always served first before my mother and me but it did not hold when there were guests.

I must explain about Vi. She was really called Violet Mary Symons – she was married to Henry Pete. They were both from Abbotskerswell village in Devon. When my mother was a teenager, Vi came to be her maid – the custom in the Dence family. Vi loved my mother dearly and when she moved to Stover, Vi went with her, first as maid and later as cook (and bottle washer). In the same way, when my mother married, Vi went with her to Highweek Rectory as cook. When John came along, she was promoted to be nanny/cook. Vi married her childhood sweetheart Henry Pete just before the Second World War. He was a sailor and petty officer, and he was immediately posted on convoy duty on a series of ships. His ship was torpedoed more than once. We children saw him as a hero whenever he turned up at our house in Plymouth on leave. He told wonderful stories of his adventures and he even took the boys and me onto his ship – a corvette – for a large meal and party. He passed us off as his own children. Vi and he never had a family of their own so we were really their adopted family. Vi stayed with Mum until she sadly died of cancer when I was in Papua. It was a great loss to us, especially to my mother as she got older.

I pressurised my parents a lot, and at thirteen years I was also sent away to board at my beloved Stover School, founded by my mother, where my Aunt Phyllis was now headmistress. How happy I was, despite missing my brothers fiercely. Our holidays were all the better for it. When we lived in Plymouth, we mostly went to North Cornwall for holidays. It was near and did not use much scarce petrol. My parents bought a very small cottage (now called *Gull Cottage*) on the cliffs of Porthcothan Bay. I still visit from time to time. We loved those beach and surfing holidays, spending many hours every day at the beach and joined by many little friends. It was really a shame that, when we moved to Salisbury, my parents felt they must sell that cottage, which is now worth thousands. In those days, petrol was impossible to obtain and very expensive so we had to change our holiday venues.

Then began our annual trek to Scotland, even further away. My father had student friends living on the west coast. He also had cousins in Northumberland, where we usually spent several cold nights in tents on our way up-country. My father had an ancient *Armstrong Siddeley* car (DYC 626).

We all crammed into it with our luggage strapped on the back. John and I, along with Vi, travelled in the back with a large Moses basket for baby Rob jammed in front of us on a case. Little Tim – he was very little then – was squashed in the front on a cushion between Mum and Dad (at the wheel). He must have been very uncomfortable but no one complained. We were too happy to upset anyone. We bought picnics on the way and enjoyed the 'lovely buns' our mother usually found everywhere. Also I saved up chocolate for the journey from our rations – there was just one shop in Salisbury where one could find chocolate bars – and we all loved it. It was strictly rationed all the holidays. Most years my father planned a working holiday. This was all he could afford for us. He used to find a parish wanting a relief priest for August – with a house for us and a small allowance for travel. We went to the Isle of Mull under this arrangement and later to Appin near Oban. Poor Dad – he had to prepare sermons, but did it cheerfully so that we could see the places he loved. I loved it too, as did Tim. I suspect John and Rob disliked the Scottish midges too much, especially when we camped. Our last family summer holidays took place on the lovely island of Raasay, off Skye, where our main occupation was walking, as well as fishing for mackerel. I was a medical student then and hated the end of the long summer holidays with my brothers.

***

I am often asked, 'When did you decide to be a doctor?' Well, I think it was all due to Great-aunt Jessie. She was my mother's aunt, a dear sister of my mother's mother, and after staying with their family for a while when my mother was a little girl, she married and went off to be a missionary in Peru – and never came back. This influenced my mother hugely and then me. Aunt Jessie died there of a fever after having her second baby, and her distraught husband – a doctor – brought the two little girls back to England by ship. My mother played with them as a child and I also met them later. When I heard the stories from my mother, my thinking was, 'Why did Aunt Jessie die? My mother did not die in childbirth – she had four of us – without a doctor. Why couldn't Aunt Jessie's doctor husband save her? I think I should do better!'

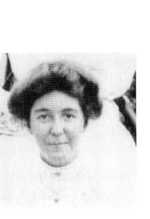
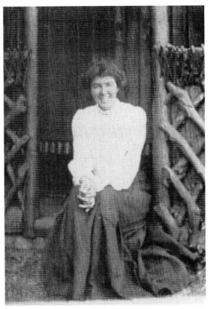

*Great-aunt Jessie*

The overseas tradition is strong in my family, with another aunt – my father's sister Winifred – working overseas as a teacher with the Colonial Service. She came to stay when on leave and she told us stories of her life, which excited me. One of my mother's sisters, Doris, was a missionary nurse in Argentina. But why did I want to be a doctor? Nursing was what most nice girls took up in my school. I remember a solemn occasion at school when my parents sat me down – with Mother's sister, the headmistress, in the room – and asked me what I intended to do with my life? Would I be a nurse or even a physiotherapist? I was horrified at the idea and quickly said, 'No! I will be a doctor.' My mother and father were very concerned. How could I do this? I would have to get a scholarship and gain entry to a London medical school – and they didn't take many girls then. My school was not happy with me. It meant I had to take A level sciences and they had no proper laboratories. I must have been a great nuisance to them – but we all managed. The school hired a physics teacher for me – every Saturday morning for two years – and I passed my A levels in the time. I also entered and obtained a Wiltshire County major scholarship for my six-year medical course.

# Auntie Gui ( correct name Winifred Joan Key)

I am adding this note as few people know or appreciate what she did. When she died of a brain tumour – quite young in today's terms – I was left all her personal belongings, including her diaries, passports, photos and letters. They were an eye-opener to me, so I have written a brief summary of her life. She trained as a teacher (classics was her subject) and in 1930 offered for the Colonial Service as a teacher. Her first posting was to a school in Georgetown, British Guyana, hence her family nickname – Gui. She was home on leave when my mother and father were married and her diaries show her concern for her father who was ailing. (Her parents lived in Aylesbeare in Devon then.) Her next posting – around 1939 – was to Malaya to a girls' secondary school in Kuala Lumpur. She loved that school and later became headmistress.

*Malay Girls' College, October 1947: Auntie Gui and the High Commissioner to Malaya*

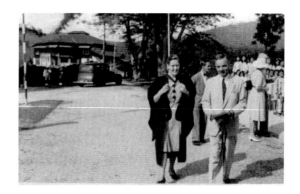

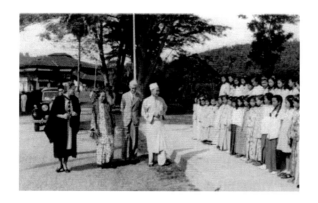

*With the Sultan of Selangur*

26

But Malaya fell to the Japanese and she had a bad time. She did not record just what happened to her and various stories were passed round the family: most likely she was in a ship that was torpedoed and she saved a child – swimming miles with the child on her back; but she never talked or wrote about it (another reason for me writing my memoirs).

The next record I have is in India, Bombay; where she arrived from where? And reported for posting. The Colonial Office in their wisdom sent her to Kenya to teach in a girls' school. I think she was very unhappy. Nobody wanted a classics teacher and her heart was back in Malaya. She wrote letters to the Colonial Office asking for transfer – but to no avail. That is, until 1944, when she was sent home and transferred back to Malaya as headmistress of her old school. She was thrilled and writes of her delight. Life is cruel sometimes. When she got out there she became ill – very ill. No one said exactly what it was but it left her with partial paralysis of her left leg and difficulty walking. To me it was clearly poliomyelitis. Many adults about that time contracted polio overseas. There was no vaccination for it then and, even at home, it was a dreaded and killing infection. There was little treatment for Gui in Malaya and she was sent home to post-war UK to recuperate.

She never did go back. She lived with our family for a while, having no home. My father and she did not get on. Father teased her constantly about her gammy leg. From her papers, I know she entered a long dispute with the Colonial Office trying to get medical help, or at least some compensation and a pension. She had many formal letters from them and several medical examinations, but they never came to a clear diagnosis and never conceded any job-related condition. The letters are full of civil-service speak and totally unsympathetic to her penniless and jobless situation. Poor Auntie Gui – what a lonely and miserable time it must have been! She never got an overseas job again, but she did manage to get a good teaching post in the UK – at Bedford Girl's High School, where she stayed until just before she died. She also trained as a Reader in the church and was heavily involved in her local church life. I wish I had known her better, but she was not easy to get close to.

By the way, for any who doubt my claim that I was to be called 'Elizabeth', in Gui's 1938 diary, she records for 26 February, 'Elizabeth Joan born.' Elizabeth was crossed through and 'Penelope' added. The entries are faint but legible.

My brothers were by this time entering university at Cambridge – one of them going to my father's old college. Another 'unfair' was echoing round my brain, but it did not matter as I was entered for Guy's Hospital as one of the statutory ten girls in a year of 120 men. I was amazed when I was accepted, at just 17 years old. What a huge transformation took place in my (so far) protected life. I lived in Hall for two years with a close group of friends, who all shared a rented flat after the second year. To this day I have remained good friends with Mary, my first room-mate in Hall. It was a really hard slog for me, I admit. We did not have much time for a social life – despite the abundance of men in our classes. I think the most social times I had were around our dissecting body in the anatomy class! I still remember my mates from then, though have lost touch with most.

I graduated as a doctor in 1961, now 23 years old. I was already thinking of distant lands, but did not know where to go or what to do there. When I was into my third medical residency at Greenbank Hospital in Plymouth, my dear Aunt Phyllis asked me to go with her to Australia to visit her brother, my Uncle Arthur. She would pay for a one-way ticket by ship. I agreed without hesitation – I just knew it was the right step for me. I trusted completely that I would find work in Australia – I had good qualifications. Little did I know that my parents were not so sure. Unknown to me, my father wrote to a friend of his who worked as a missionary priest in Papua. I had heard of him and even met him once when he was home on leave.

There was a big crowd of family and friends to see us off at the docks, and I had no idea how long I would be away. I knew I would miss my brothers hugely, especially my 'little' brother Robbie, who was growing up fast. The sea journey from Tilbury Docks to Melbourne took six long weeks. My memories of the voyage are not very happy. Aunt Phyllis was still my 'headmistress' and she was a very formal person. She was happy as we were seated at the First Officer's table – not the Captain's, thank goodness! Phyl spent many hours walking the deck, while I preferred to join deck games. I did not really enjoy the evening social events, especially not knowing people much. I think we played 'Bingo' but I hated it. The best part of the journey were the stopovers. We went through the Red Sea and I was fascinated by the desert and all the fishing boats. I did not get off in Aden – I think I was too scared. But we landed in Colombo in Ceylon, and visited the hills and tea plantations.

On docking in Melbourne, I was very surprised to have an air-letter presented to me – from Henry Kendall (Archdeacon of Papua). He asked me to consider travelling at once to Papua – by air – to take the vacant position of locum medical officer for four months at the Eroro Mission Hospital. What an excitement! I knew it was my calling and I cabled, 'Yes – send me a ticket.' I was taken on for four months and stayed in Papua New Guinea (PNG) for *eleven years*.

After visiting Uncle Arthur, and a little time to see something of Australia, we drove to Canberra to meet a few of the Aussie relatives, especially Ann Robson and the family, then I had to fly from Sydney – my first flight ever. I was terrified and thought the plane was on fire when the engines started – there were no jets then, they were all propeller planes. I was comforted by a missionary sitting next to me who was more worried about the large cake in her bag that she was taking to her colleagues, who never had cake to eat. We duly arrived at Port Moresby airport in the very early hours of a September morning in 1962.

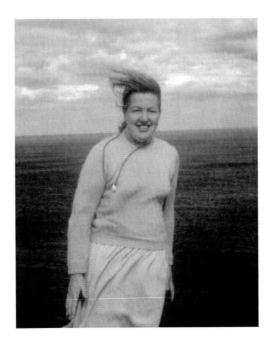

*Pene travelling in Australia*

# Chapter 2: Papua New Guinea – My formative years

Then, in 1962, my adventures began. I registered with the health authorities as locum Medical-Officer-in-Charge, St Margaret's Anglican Mission Hospital, Eroro. I don't remember, but I must have had some inkling that I would work overseas – or I would not have brought my medical registration papers with me. Anyway, I had them and all was well.

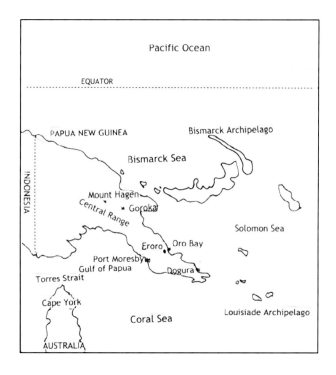

*Papua New Guinea map*

## The start

I had no idea what to expect. Geography had not been a strong subject of mine. I thought 'the natives' would live in grass houses and wear little – but had few other ideas. For my first few days and nights I stayed at the mission transit house in Port Moresby, run by the Franciscan Order of Friars. I was introduced to gecko lizards, and to tropical vegetables and fruits, and shown the shanty towns of Hanuabada, as well as the port. Then early one morning I flew over the central mountain range to Oro Bay. Our ancient DC3 aeroplane circled lazily over a makeshift airstrip, and after landing noisily, the pilot muttered, 'There's no one there.' I climbed out, with the mailbag. But still no one to meet us and I was getting worried. The pilot decided he had to go on. He would leave me – but not the mailbag, as there was no one to sign for it. I remedied that fast – I had been eyeing the mailbag hungrily during the flight as I was hoping for a letter from home. Then, just as I was preparing myself for a wait in the middle of nowhere in the mounting tropical heat, we heard – and then saw – a jeep, swaying dangerously towards us down the runway. Everyone said, 'That's Father Jeremy.' Indeed it was. Like many early missionaries there, he was English, and only he would drive a jeep as fast as that down an airstrip made of iron Marsden matting (left over from the war). He introduced himself and welcomed me, seized the mailbag and signalled for me to climb in. This was the first of many precarious jeep rides I had. It is one of the most uncomfortable and unsafe means of transport I know – at least, for the passengers in the back. It's all right for the driver. So I arrived at St Margaret's mission station and hospital, where I lived and worked for four months.

## Oro Bay

Eroro was the village name. It was about three miles inland from Oro Bay, on the northern Papuan coast, almost opposite Port Moresby. Now the hospital has been moved to Oro Bay itself, where it is more convenient for the many patients who arrive there by canoe and ship. I was shown the doctor's house, where I was to sleep. We all ate together at the Mission House, looked after by young housegirls from the village.

I was terrified alone in the house at first. I was unprepared for the teeming insect life from the bush which came up close to the house. I had got used to the geckos in Port Moresby, but here I encountered spiders, centipedes and scorpions early on – to be followed quickly by snakes: grass snakes and the infamous Papuan Black Snake, which regularly killed its victims. I remember the night sounds of the tropical creatures, with particularly noisy frogs – and there were crocodiles in the sea and river at Oro Bay.

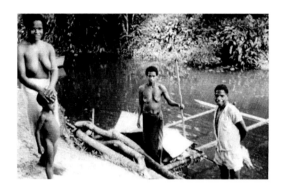

*Local transport*

The hospital surprised me. I suppose I was expecting something a bit more substantial with better basic facilities because it was built and belonged to the Mission and had been started there about ten years before. But it was very basic. There were four wards: concrete floors and straw walls and roof – no beds. There was an out-patient department that was always full, and an operating theatre and ancient X-ray. What an experience!

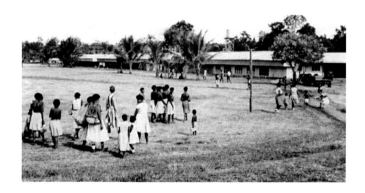

*St Margaret's Hospital, Eroro*

I will always be in debt to the two Mission Sisters – one English and one Australian, trained midwives both, who introduced me to my work very kindly, trying to make up for my ignorance of basic tropical medicine and

32

tropical diseases of the kind I had to treat at once. I think I learned fast – especially how to 'make do' with what was available in the way of medicines and equipment. I had to learn from them how to administer an ether anaesthetic, using a face mask and gauze – and dropping the ether to make the patient sleep; and to shoot and develop my own X-rays, using an ancient machine run on a small generator which I had first to start up. The mission station boasted electricity for four hours every evening: the rest of the time it was run on special request only, such as when doing emergency operations – usually Caesarean sections.

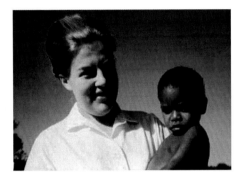

*An early photo of me as a missionary doctor in Papua New Guinea*

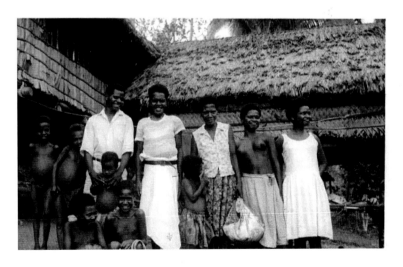

*An aid-post orderly in a mountain village*

33

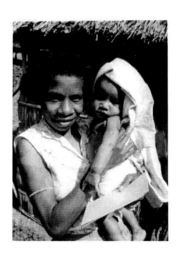

*Medical assistant's wife and child*

The prevalent diseases there were diarrhoea in children, malaria and tuberculosis – and then there were emergency obstetrics. Thinking back, my most memorable patients were quadruplets, born on a canoe out in the bay – or rather, I delivered the fourth on dry land. Their mother was stoical and took it all more calmly than us. The biggest multiple birth I had cared for was triplets – in England. Sadly, the only babe that survived this time was the fourth. The first three got too cold on the canoe. It is easy for us to assume that no one gets cold in the tropical heat. But a cool breeze on the sea and no coverings can quickly chill a tiny newborn too much for survival. Multiple births are very common in Papua: it has been shown that as many as one in eighty births is a multiple – mostly twins. There is no great stigma attached to twins as I later learned is the case in parts of India and Africa, where the second twin child is considered an evil spirit.

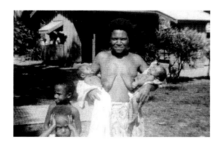

*Oro Bay: twins*

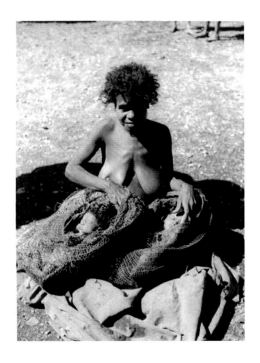

*More twins*

Another new experience was the medical radio session. Ahead of its time, the mission had established radio networks at all the outlying missions, most of which had health posts run by nurses or medical orderlies. Every day, one of the mission doctors sat by the radio two or three times to answer questions or advise staff and medical orderlies on any difficult cases they had. I enjoyed this new challenge. I frequently operated the schedule by myself and appreciated being able to support our professional staff in this way. Many of the staff were Australian, but once they got used to my 'very English voice', it seemed that they appreciated my input and consulted me more. These medical radio sessions were a great help to mission families, especially wives, who were bringing up their families in the remote interior, far from medical help. We devised a medical box for all these families so that we knew exactly what medicines were available when we gave advice. It was still heartbreaking to hear of a very ill baby or child and trying to help the mother fighting for a tiny life, when treatment would have been simple if we had had the child in hospital.

Occasionally we were able to commission the 'St Gabriel', the mission aeroplane for an emergency air evacuation. Can you imagine what these words meant to a panic-stricken mother: 'St Gabriel landing in ten minutes'? We were not always so lucky and, as has happened to many missionary families all over the world, a tiny grave was left behind.

## The Managalas Mountains

One of the nurses, Nancy, became a good friend and she introduced me to the world of 'patrols' – we went out to villages, near and far, on foot, by jeep and by canoe.

We always sent word ahead by radio or by runners that we were coming. In each village we set up a clinic to see every child, give immunisations, nutrition advice and treatment for anyone ill. As we extended our outreach into the mountains behind Oro Bay, we found more and more problems: congenital defects, polio, leprosy, tuberculosis and skin diseases among the children, who had had no contact with health services. We were certainly the first white women they had ever seen and we enjoyed their cheerful friendliness and even their curiosity. I spent many rewarding days and weeks on patrol in the Managalas Mountains.

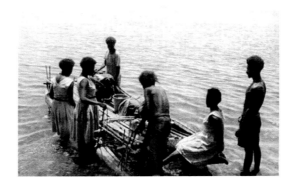

*A patrol canoe: I sat at the front end on the right, with the packs on the outrigger on the left. Here, others are having a lift before we leave*

*Nancy and a
student nurse*

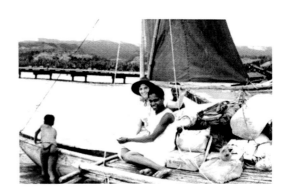

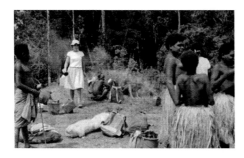

*Sister Pat with village
women*

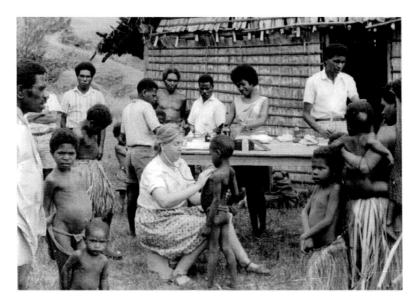

*Inland patrol clinic. Lancelot is at the table at the back while I
examine a child with a cough*

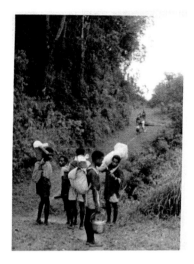

*A line of carriers on our patrol*

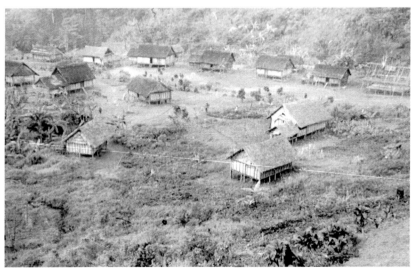

*A mission station in the Managalas*

There was a small bush hospital at the mission station, often with many patients and a wide range of illnesses. There was a mission priest, medical orderlies, teachers and a school full of children needing a lot of healthcare, and I sometimes went for two or three weeks to help out – and from there patrolled deep into the interior. The scenery was magnificent: virgin jungle full of birds of paradise, hornbills and even cassowary (which could bite viciously). One memorable day when on the radio schedule at Dogura, I was contacted from the Managalas about a child who had been bitten on the abdomen by a cassowary. Its beak had gone deep and there was bowel protruding. We evacuated her to our hospital by plane but we could not save her. We all had a big respect for the bird after that. The other tragic cases we found there often included serious burns – especially affecting little girls who, from about four years old, were dressed in grass skirts. Because of the cold up in the mountains, families huddled around open fires inside their grass houses in the evening and at night. Little girls in grass skirts could get too close to the flames and their skirts would go up in flames. I remember finding a girl of about seven with deep burns all down her trunk and legs. We tried to save her but she was too deeply shocked and our treatment away from the hospital too basic, so we lost her.

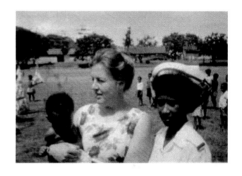

*Sister Leah and me at a mission station*

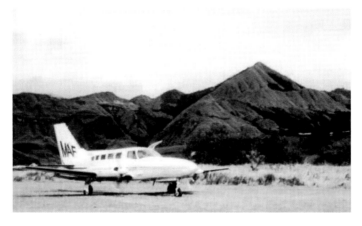

*The 'St Gabriel'*

I must introduce you better to one means of transport in those early years – the mission aeroplane – aptly named St Gabriel, a single-engine Cessna plane operated by MAF (Missionary Aviation Fellowship) for the diocese. I first met it at Eroro, where I and my team needed to be lifted in and out of the Managalas Mountains – or otherwise make a journey of twelve hours by canoe and then three days' hike uphill. Getting a ride in the little monoplane cut the journey to ten minutes from the grass airstrip at the mission station to a rough mountain strip carved out of the jungle. It was a nerve-wracking experience to fly up there. First the plane had to take off over the coconut trees – much prized by the local villagers. One terrible day for me was when a new pilot failed to take off and instead played dodgems with the trees – not actually hitting any but stopping in a hole and having to be rescued by the mission tractor – to start the journey again. This time we took off safely and made the long sweep out over Oro Bay and turned inland towards the mountain ridge. The pilot turned to me beside him and asked, 'Do you know the way?' just as if we were going to the corner shop. I rather weakly replied, 'I think so. You go between those two ridges.' We climbed slowly and crept towards the ridge – then from the white-faced pilot: 'I don't think we will clear it like this – too heavy! I must turn round now or we will bump it.' this was followed by the nerve-wracking steep turn and a try at a slightly lower ridge – mercifully clearing it. We were delighted to see the tiny mission airstrip on the slopes of the mountain below us. There was only one way to land – uphill into the mountain – easy! But take-offs were downhill, hoping we would clear the gully at the downhill end. It was a steep slope and the load was strictly limited. One good friend, Father Doug, made a practice of kneeling on the airstrip whenever the St Gabriel arrived and, with all the people, praying loudly for a safe take-off or landing. I'm sure the Lord heard him, but we, on board, did not feel much confidence in this non-technical approach.

*A child with TB at Embi*

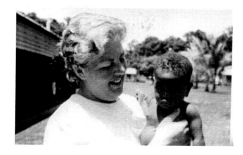

I loved it all. The four months went fast and I was invited to visit the nearby TB and Leprosy Hospital, St Luke's, at Embi.

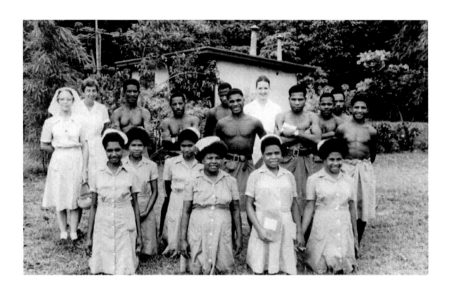

*Hospital staff at Embi: Sister Nance and Dorothy at left*

The legendary, long-serving mission doctor, Blanche Biggs (an Australian), was going on furlough – would I stand in for her for eight months? There was nothing I wanted more. I accepted. But how little I knew about these two diseases – and there were 250-300 inpatients suffering from them. Again I learned fast, first from Dr Biggs before she left and then from the two nursing sisters. I often sought help from the now-returned doctor, Maurice Dowell, at Eroro. Patients were sent to Embi from a wide area of Papua, from both government and mission hospitals. It was officially a government hospital but run by the Anglican mission, which supplied the staff. Patients usually stayed from nine months to two years – a long-term business. As leprosy was fast dying out at that time, we had few new patients admitted – just lots of very chronic patients. They were ostracised by their families, poverty-stricken and very miserable. Most of the patients were extremely poor but at least they got three meals a day in our care and many made a good recovery – though not all. My introduction in Embi gave me a good grounding in the treatment of these two debilitating diseases, which was to stand me in good stead when I took charge of another leprosarium in Africa at a later date.

It was here at Embi that I met the Haste family, who became lifelong friends, and their youngest daughter Clare, who was born later, became my godchild. Bob and Rosemary were mission staff from the UK. They arrived with two small children and another on the way – greatly adding to my responsibilities. Bob, who later became a priest, was then the hospital maintenance man – very much needed and valued by all of us. He could get us out of most problems as well as keeping the electric generator running for us. He also provided me with one of my most taxing emergencies. One day he ran the tractor (used for cutting grass) over himself – dislocating his hip and traumatising his back. I knew I was not strong enough to reduce that hip joint – so I sent the tractor (our only transport apart from bicycles) the four miles to Eroro to fetch Dr Dowell – who came and helped me first anaesthetise and then reduce the dislocation. Poor Bob was confined to his bed for three months at our hospital. I don't know to this day how he managed to put up with the rather crude nursing and medical care we gave him – but he did, and he walked again and was back at work in six months – cared for by his loving family, now with one addition, baby Mark (who is now a nurse with the flying doctor service in Darwin). Bob had that hip replaced in later life – the damage, I'm sure, a legacy of those days.

Other patients I remember at Embi included dear Magdalene, a 17-year-old girl with severe tuberculosis of the lungs. One day she collapsed with chest pain and shortness of breath. I had read up my TB by now – so I knew she had a pneumothorax (air in the chest cavity). I knew that I must insert a big needle to release the trapped air – if she was to survive. This was my first, but not last, time of doing such a procedure. She made a good recovery and went on to marry one of our medical orderlies; they later became leaders in the church – Magdalene was President of the Mothers' Union, in which role she visited me in the UK later. I often gave thanks that I was given the skill and knowledge to treat her successfully. (I also used to train the medical orderlies, many of them coming straight to us from school.)

Dot and Nance were my two fellow staff at Embi – along with Bob. Dot managed the store and ran the feeding of all patients. My memory is of her standing in the hatch to the kitchen, spooning out rice, fresh vegetables, meat and tinned fish three times a day to hungry patients. Their diet was a major component of their care and treatment. It had to be good, and Dot spent much time buying fresh food from local people in exchange for salt and tobacco. Nance was a nursing sister and, like Dot, was from Australia. She had long experience of the mission and had worked up and down the country. I learned a huge amount from her. She taught the student nurses and we relied on them to care for any bed patients – though most were up and about. I valued Nance's experience and wise head in clinical matters. She understood better than most that a very raw young doctor needed a bit of help and advice at times. I was only in my mid-twenties then.

One memorable afternoon Father Jeremy arrived on the tractor. He called to me, 'Pene, get up behind me on the tractor. Your mother wants to speak to you urgently on the radio.' Indeed, it was just possible to contact home by tele-radio and I had told my parents how they could do this in emergency only. So I feared the worst as I clung to the tractor and Jeremy, and bounced down the three miles of track between Eroro and Embi. When I reached the radio hut, I could just make out my mother's voice sounding far, far away. I interrupted her with, 'Hello Mum; what is the matter?' Down the line came: 'Nothing – I just wanted to talk to you!' Complete horror and disbelief on all the faces around me. What a waste of precious radio time – and petrol. Mum said later that she just had to hear my voice as it was so long (over a year) since we spoke. She did not understand what her call meant to us there. It took a long time for me to live that one down, though it was very nice to hear her.

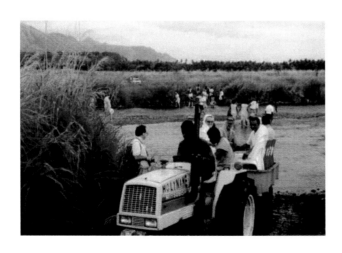

*River crossing with the mission tractor transport*

43

Dr Biggs returned from furlough ready to pick up the reins again and I had to look around for work. I was not yet ready to leave PNG . Out of the blue, I received a letter from the Bishop (David Hand) asking if I would become a permanent member of staff, based as mission doctor at Dogura – the mission head station, to the south east of Eroro. I had to think long and hard. The term of duty would be five years without leave and medically I would be completely alone. Dogura's only access to the outside world was a monthly ship and occasional stops by the St Gabriel. Then I was very aware of the gaps in my knowledge of tropical diseases, by which I was surrounded. So I negotiated with the Bishop. I said yes, I would come on condition they supported me for a short course in tropical medicine first. He agreed – apparently readily – and I was enrolled for the diploma course in tropical diseases at Sydney University, with board and lodging at the House of the Epiphany – the Anglican Mission training centre. I was to start term in February 1964, and allowed home leave before returning for my five-year term. It was considered generous in those days. My salary would be £75 per year, with accommodation and food all found.

## First Visit to the Highlands

The only problem with all these arrangements was that it was November and my course in Australia started in February; where would I stay in the interim? Another offer came from the Mission. Would I go to the Highlands for three months to help out at Movi mission hospital? They had no doctor.

There began a series of adventures in the New Guinea Highlands. I travelled to Lae in a violent thunderstorm in an old DC3 aircraft – we were overloaded as usual. Adult passengers sat facing each other round the plane. The centre was filled with cargo. Every adult had a child on their lap – some quite big. The plane bucked and bumped as it was struck by lightning and heavy rain. Most children and many adults were airsick. It was terrifying. We made it to Lae airport – a proper tarmac runway seemed a gift from heaven. I was met and put up at the rectory overnight. The next day we boarded another small old plane – destination Goroka, capital of the Highlands. From Goroka it was a short plane journey to another mission airstrip at a place called Nambiufa, in a village about six miles' walk from

Movi station. I got to know that walk (climb) well in my time there.

Movi is a most beautiful place nestling in a valley with high mountains (6-7,000 ft) all around. The people live in villages mostly on mountain ridges (for security) and have to climb down to the river valleys – thousands of feet down and up – to fetch water. Children abounded and were never far from us strange white people as we walked or slowly climbed the five-mile track.

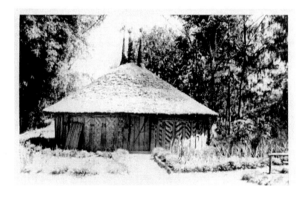

*A traditional highland roundhouse*

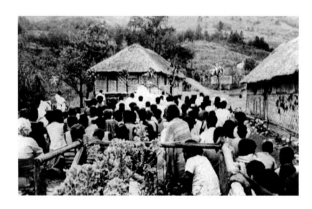

*Going to church at the mission station at Movi*

I was introduced to the small bush hospital by a very experienced and efficient nurse who had looked after the work for many years on her own. Bridget clearly did not relish my entrance on the scene. What could I offer that she could not do? I see her point now – the days of nurse-practitioners were far away then (the 1960s) and she had such experience. However, I did what I could and took on the patrolling work which she found hard –

walking many miles in the incredibly wild and mountainous countryside, where the sun shone endlessly but where it was really cold at night. When we went out like this, we usually had local village men to act as porters and guides to the next village. We would pay them in goods, bartering – usually with salt and tobacco. We would also have a medical orderly with us, but we did not expect violence, although the people were wild Highlanders – often in feather headdresses and wearing strings of bone or wood round their necks, depicting the number of men each had killed. They were awesome to encounter – and curious about us. Tribal fights were all too common and their custom of pay-back killing was very hard to break. I learned more of this in a later posting in the Highlands.

We had a marvellous Christmas at Movi – with enormous services in the new bush church. The people dressed in their traditional finery and brought pigs to cook and eat, along with the traditional Mu-mu (root vegetables buried in the ground with hot stones to cook them). There was fantastic dancing all afternoon and evening – a time to remember for ever.

*Pictures from Movi:*

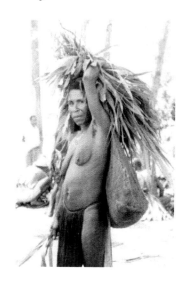 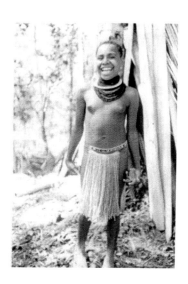

*A typical Siane woman, carrying firewood,*    *A young Highland girl*

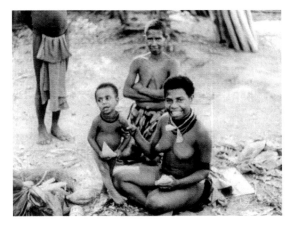

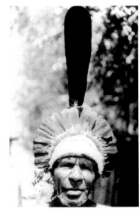

*Three generations*

*An old Highland man*

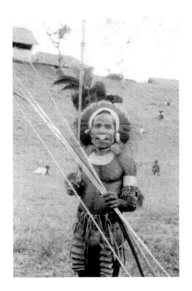

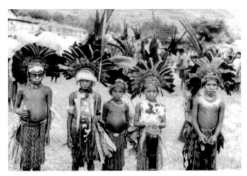

*Siane children dressed for a feast,
Christmas 1964*

*Highland chieftain*

I left Movi in late January for Sydney and my studies. What I remember most was the bitter cold when the Sydney winter arrived after a few months. I had come from the tropical heat and was without suitable clothes. I had no warm clothes at all and no money either. My mission stipend of £75 per annum would not run to a new coat. So I made friends, and when I turned up at someone's house for lunch or dinner, wearing only a cotton dress, they invariably offered to lend me warm clothes – and that is how I managed. I returned them all when I left.

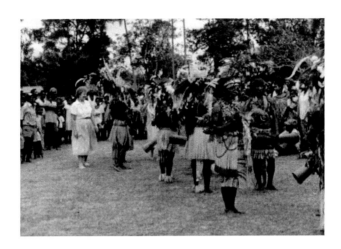

*On a later visit, with Managalas dancers for a celebration*

So my time at the 'House of Epiphany' in Sydney was significant to the development of my faith and developing friendships for life. All the students there were training like me – but to be missionaries. We had a strict routine of chapel every morning before going to work. Then the other students went to their lectures, while I walked to the university for my own lectures. I enjoyed the course and met interesting doctors who, like me, were en route to the tropics, but they were not all missionaries. It served its purpose and my subsequent knowledge of tropical diseases stood me in good stead all my working life in the tropics.

A great bonus for me at that time was getting to know my Australian relations. Sadly, my Uncle Arthur had by now died. I got to know my elderly cousin, Agnes Dence, who had visited my parents in England several times. She was daughter to my Great-uncle John, who had left England at the age of 15 to seek his fortune in Australia. He achieved this and founded a prolific branch of our family living in and around Sydney. The family that were especially good to me were the Robsons: Ann Robson (née Dence) was married to a surgeon and living in Canberra. They had a large family with whom I made friends and I still visit them when in Australia.

Sadly, my cousin Agnes died in 2007, aged 106. She was a true Dence, looking very like my Aunt Phyllis and my Grandmother Dence, who I may resemble too.

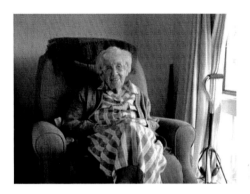

*My cousin Agnes at 101*

I was there for nine months, and as I have said, made wonderful friends at the House of the Epiphany, among an annual intake of around twenty missionaries-in-training. I studied hard and achieved my Diploma in Tropical Medicine, feeling much better equipped for the next phase of my life in Papua. But I went home first – to England, my parents and my three brothers, all now finishing their studies, starting careers and getting married. It was difficult to leave them for my five-year term, but I was young and resilient and had a great love for my work. I felt valued and needed where I was going and I went with my family's blessing; although I think my brothers thought I was slightly mad.

***

The following is taken from a report in my parents' local newspaper under the title:

## 'Bishop's daughter reports from mission hospital in Papua'
A vivid picture of life at the Anglican Mission Station at Dogura, in far-off Papua, where she is the doctor in charge of St. Barnabas Hospital, has been sent home to Truro by Dr. Penelope Key, only daughter of the Bishop of Truro and Mrs. Key.

Before returning to Dogura early in January, Dr. Penelope Key was commissioned to her adventurous task as a medical missionary in Papua and New Guinea by her father at morning service in Truro Cathedral. Many well-wishers in Cornwall, following an appeal letter, gave their practical support in money and gifts for the purchase of urgently needed hospital equipment.

Dr. Key wrote her first report from a little village high up in the mountains behind Dogura called Wanama on a patrol to examine all babies and children under five, to see sick people, to treat them, or send them down to the main hospital, and to help and encourage the out-station medical orderlies.

NEW HOSPITAL

Dr. Key said it had been decided that the present St. Barnabas Hospital must be moved to a new site, where development could occur without fear of overcrowding and where they could be sure of good water supplies and drainage. St. Barnabas would continue to be the only hospital in a district with a population of 17,500.

"My practice is truly a 'general' one. One minute I am taking out teeth or stitching lacerations, while the next I am treating some exotic tropical disease or operating on a rare tumour.

"From a medical angle the field is vast, and there is enough to keep six doctors busy every minute of the day."

\*\*\*

I arrived in September 1965 in Port Moresby and thence to Dogura (for four years), by way of our mission ship the *MV Maclaren King* (named after a famous missionary). This was the first of many journeys aboard her. It was a spectacular voyage up the Milne Bay coast to Wedau Pier – the port for Dogura – or rather the beach where we disembarked with our luggage.

There was a warm welcome from the Bishop (Bishop John Chisholm) and the nursing staff, who had managed alone for some months, waiting for their new doctor to arrive. This time I did not feel so ignorant – and armed with my new knowledge and books, I set to work.

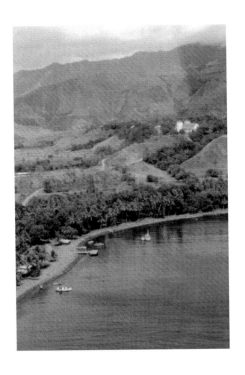

*Wedau pier*

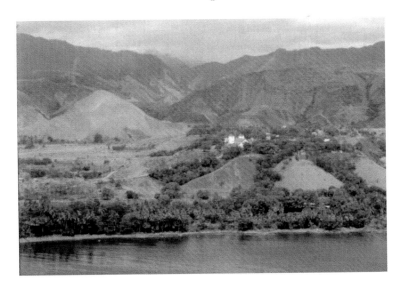

*Dogura Mission – my house is among the trees on the right*

# The Mission

The mission community of perhaps a hundred became all-important to me. It included the mission priests (expatriate and Papuan); the theological training college; the teacher training college, St Aidan's; the Holy Name Girls' Secondary School and St Paul's Primary School, as well as the nurses' training school, St Bartholomew's, and the hospital. The staff of these institutions all had some paid expatriates, many Papuan mission staff and some volunteers – British VSOs (Voluntary Service Overseas) and Australians AVAs (Australian Volunteers Abroad). We were under the supervision of the head of station – Bishop John. The only set rules concerned attendance at cathedral services. We were expected at Holy Communion (Mass) every morning at 6.30 am. It was not compulsory, but just expected – so most of us turned up and learned to love it. Sunday morning service was a definite 'must'. The cathedral was marvellous inside and on Sundays it was filled with Wedau villagers and their large families, all sitting on mats on the concrete floor, singing in harmony in their Wedau language. The service and sermon were in Wedauan, the local language which we all had to learn, and lasted a good three hours – and we sat on the ground too – women on the left side and men on the right. (The Wedau language was not difficult: it had originally been spoken only, and when recorded in script, this was done phonetically, so it was easy to read aloud, to sing, and indeed, fairly easy to learn.) I used to welcome medical calls during service, and must admit to pre-arranging them on occasions! And the radio schedule quite often interrupted a long service for me.

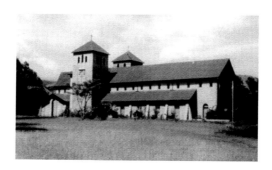

*Dogura Cathedral of St Peter and St Paul*

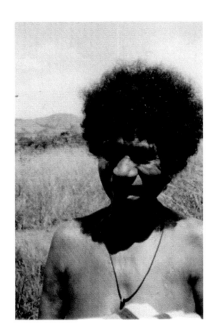

*A typical Wedauan woman, Mrs Kibikibi, who later became Mothers' Union President*

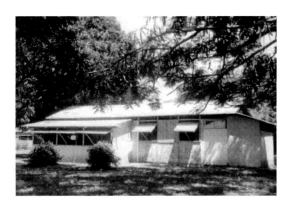

*My house – Tavara*

We all ate together in the main Dogura mission house nearby. We had a mission cook/housekeeper, Jocelyn, who fed us well on the limited fresh food available to us locally. Jocelyn was a good friend to all of us. She lived with her family (two small children) in a tiny house next to mine. The teachers all lived in the mission house, which some found very trying after a bit. Unlike me, they had little privacy. We had no electricity most of the time. We became adept at reading by pressure lamp and cooking with Primus stoves. Our needs were simple: we would spend our 'pocket money' allowance on things like postage and soap or small gifts from the Trade Store, which was run by the Mission, and most things there came from Australia. Our toilets were pit latrines outside the house and we washed in bucket showers – warm if we could get hold of a kettle of hot water. I learned to enjoy my bucket shower. I had a house-girl to clean my house and wash my clothes – a privilege of my position as doctor. I slept under a large mosquito net – there were many mosquitoes and malaria was very common.

## My house (Tavara)

The doctor before me had lived very happily in this small bungalow. It had two small bedrooms, a bathroom, a sitting room and a kitchen. It was constructed of woven grass walls, a corrugated iron roof and concrete floors. It had big windows which were open to the weather and any passing animals and people (the path to the teacher training college went down the hill on which my house stood) and it was located on a prime site on Tavara Point, from where you could look out to sea up and down the coast.

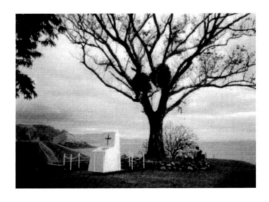

*Tavara Point, with its historic tree, where the first mission church was established, which my house overlooked*

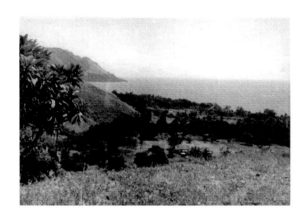

*The view from Tavara Point*

The view was marvellous and everyone was jealous of me. When I arrived at Dogura mission station, most people thought that, because I was a single woman, I would not want to live alone at Tavara. But I wanted it more than anything. I'm not sure where they planned for me to go – possibly the nurses' home or Dogura House with all the single teachers. I stuck out for my position and set about clearing Tavara of the previous occupant's left-behinds. I took up residence and set up my large mosquito net over my bed, established my study in a corner of the sitting area and a chair outside from which to gaze at the view. It spoiled me for views in the future! I did baulk at cooking while I worked full time but was able to eat *en famille* with the rest of the staff. I bought a bicycle to connect me with the hospital – only a three-minute walk away. My large bicycle, basket on the front, became a local sight as I often transported babies and small children in it.

*Myself and a local child*

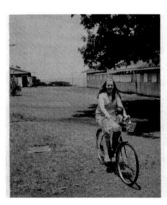

## St Barnabas Hospital

This was the first mission hospital to be built and it had much better buildings and facilities than Eroro or any others I saw. The original building was wooden and had a small delivery room, pharmacy, X-ray room and out-patient department, through which all patients passed. Mornings saw schoolchildren lined up on specially designed leg-treatment boards to have their tropical ulcers dressed. Any small injury usually went septic and quickly ulcerated. It was really difficult to clear them up in both adults and children. We had to work hard on the expatriate staff to prevent them from developing ulcers – often caused by mosquito bites.

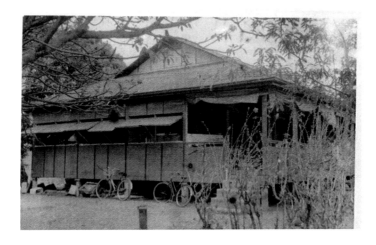

*St Barnabas Hospital*

There were four good wards each holding ten to twenty beds and often floor mats also occupied. Wards included adult surgical and medical, children's and maternity. All patients had their relatives with them, usually sleeping on a mat by their bed. So it was crowded – especially the children's ward where Mum, Dad and Granny usually all came. We tried to provide every bed with a mosquito net, but the people were not used to them and usually just lay on them. It is quite hot and airless to sleep under a net in the tropics. The operating theatre was a new building – well designed, and my pride and joy. I spent a lot of time there.

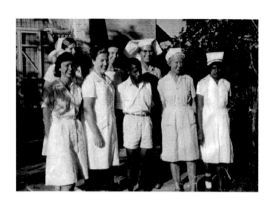

*Colleagues at
St Barnabas
Hospital,
Dogura 1968*

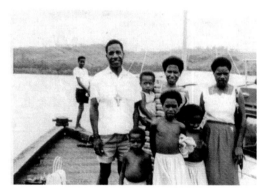

*Friends – Bishop
George and
Marcella Ambo
with some of their
family*

## The Nurses' Training School

Around thirty young girls were admitted to this school every year. It was hard to gain entry as it was a prestigious school with an excellent name all over Papua. The national government delighted in poaching St Barnabas trained nurses. The training was ward-based, the trainees working on the wards while they learned. They were our workforce in all areas. Gradually we were allowed to employ more trained nurses for the hospital and the outreach work, but money was short and we had to justify any new posts. One of the nurses we trained then is now the country's chief nursing officer and one can find St Barnabas nurses all over the country. Of course, they also made very good wives and mothers. The trainee nurses were highly popular with the male students at the two training colleges (teacher and theological).

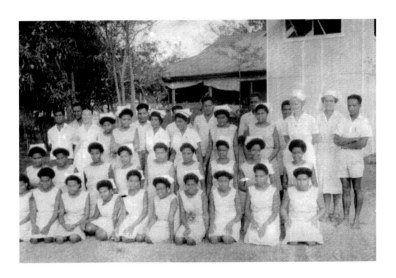

*The Nurses' Training School, 1967. Sister tutors Jean Henderson and Joan Durdin at the back.*

Because maternal health was so neglected, we quite often had orphan babies brought in for rearing. Most had fathers waiting to take them home when weaned, but some were left a long time with us and we became very attached to these gorgeous babies. I had my own special little girl, who we discovered was totally deaf. I do not know how she fared later in life, but it would have been very hard as there were no services for deaf children anywhere there.

## Policies and Plans

Early in my tenure, no doubt inspired by my course, I was determined to develop plans and policies for our work. But there was so much work every day, and so many sick patients, that there was little time to sit still and think, discuss and plan.

The decision we had to take at once was whether to concentrate our staff resources on the hospital work or keep up the extensive patrolling into the villages. We couldn't manage both without wearing out our staff. The hospital had been without a doctor for several months and patient numbers had dropped as the word got around. I felt that our priority should be to

58

build up the hospital work to provide high-quality care to those who did reach us, but at the same time we should plan a very regular series of patrols, concentrating on the remoter villages where there was most sickness. It was imperative, anyway, that we taught our nurse trainees how to undertake these visits and what to do. It was difficult at first for me to walk away from a full hospital for one to three weeks, leaving our trained nurses to manage as before, but I did. This plan was reversed in my years three to five, as referrals became more frequent and more serious. I just had to be on hand at the referral hospital, especially for maternity cases. This really was the beginning of a sort of nurse-practitioner system, with an increasing number of Papuan nurses. We appointed the first local Sisters, who were excellent. We were very proud of our mission sisters who later became leaders in the country.


## Patrolling

Our immediate surrounding population, within easy walking distance of hospital-based out-patient clinics, was about 20,000 in four big villages nearby. However, our catchment's population was nearly 100,000 scattered along the coast and inland for many miles. Out there we did not measure distances in miles – rather in walking hours. As I have said, I had discovered that ten hours' walking in the hills was covered by ten minutes flying in a light aircraft, though there were few landing strips. Most visits to coastal villages were made by boat. Occasionally we were able to use the St George motor launch, which even had one cabin for tired walkers or sick people. But it had a roll and the sea could be rough in the sound. I have rolled my way to and from outlying villages, laden with people and trusting that we would make it home.

There were two mission stations where there were expatriate nurses posted whom I tried to visit for support and medical referrals on a regular basis. I also had close touch with them by radio network, which operated the same way as at Eroro. I did a radio session three times daily – but it was all so public. Everyone else knew when one person was ill. This was rather hard on expatriate women who wanted to discuss very personal healthcare with me, but it was better than nothing and the alternative was a twelve-hour boat trip to visit me.

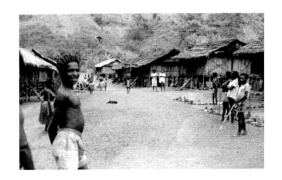

*Wonama village
main street,
inland Dogura*

*Clinic on patrol*

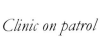

*Health centre with waiting mothers*

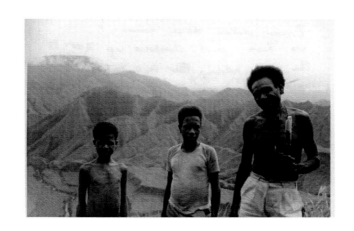

*Mountain villagers*

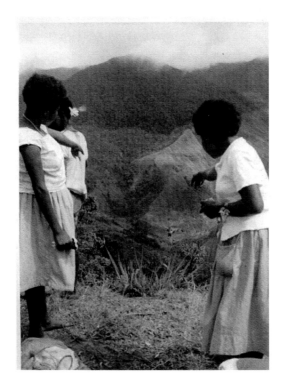

*Our Papuan sister Dorothea,*
*on patrol high in the mountains in the Denova region*

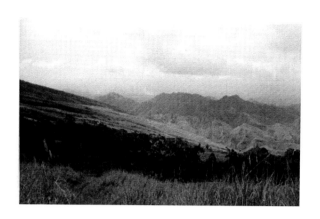

*Mountains behind Dogura*

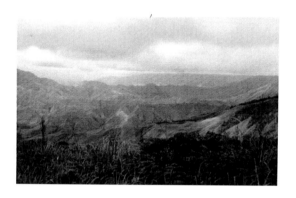

*Inland view on patrol behind Dogura*

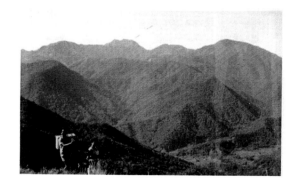

*Mountains we crossed in Denova*

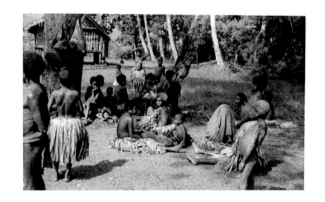

*Villagers waiting for clinic in Denova*

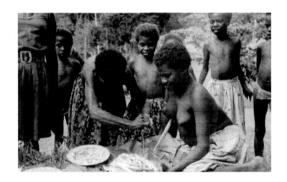

*Infant welfare clinic in Denova*

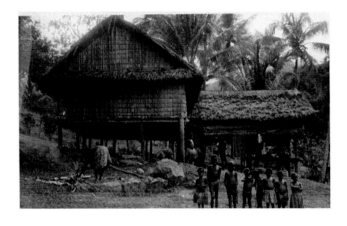

*Village houses high on stilts in Denova*

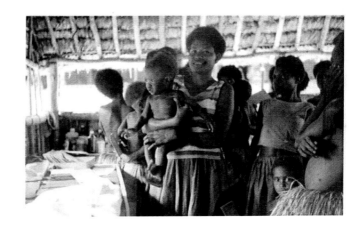

*Village clinic*

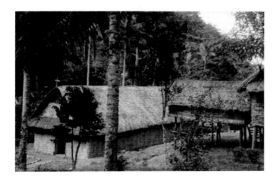

*The village church*

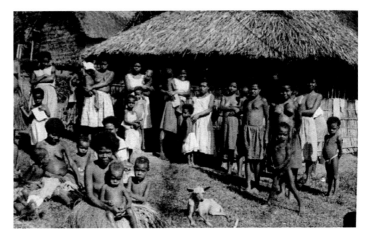

*Mothers with babies and children
gathering round our medical team on patrol*

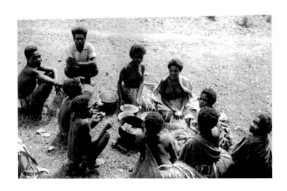

*Cooking dinner in the village*

Then there was the St Gabriel, our single-engine Cessna plane, which I have already described. Depending on the Dogura mission station budget, I was permitted to charter the plane occasionally to airlift me and my medical team (usually two trainee nurses, a trained sister and a medical assistant) to the starting-place of a patrol in the mountains. There was a new mission area called the Daga, staffed by a well-known English missionary priest and his elderly mother. They were very keen to improve healthcare in their villages and to establish aid posts staffed by trained orderlies.

I am proud now of the healthcare work we started there. We were ahead of our time – ahead of the global primary healthcare movement, initiated at Alma Ata in the USSR in 1978, and even ahead of China's barefoot doctors. In 1968 in PNG, we were training Primary Health workers – then called Aid-Post orderlies – to take essential primary healthcare to their own people in the villages. The health posts were built by the local communities in the place they chose as central to most people. Occasionally, they sent men or women to be trained at the Mission and then return to run the aid post in their village.

## Dogura 1968 Royal Visit

At this time, we had a diverting interlude. The Anglican Mission, through the Australian Board of Missions (ABM), had nurtured a link between the

Papuan church high school for boys, the Martyrs' Memorial School (MMS) and Geelong Grammar School outside Melbourne. The latter was the school chosen by the Queen and Prince Philip to finish schooling their eldest son, Charles. Then a young man of seventeen or eighteen, he entered into the life of the school with enthusiasm. The school took their link with MMS seriously and in 1966 arranged an exchange visit for some of their senior pupils with seniors at MMS. There was great excitement when we heard that their party included Prince Charles, but even more when we learned that Dogura would also feature in their itinerary. The group would stay with us on the mission station for several days and each of us were to prepare a programme of activities to demonstrate our work.

I was only marginal to the detailed planning, which must have been a nightmare for our leaders. I had to submit my own detailed CV to Buckingham Palace to determine whether I could be trusted to provide HRH with a reasonable medical service should he need it. I was flattered to be approved (by radio) and was called upon during the royal visit.

My staff and I planned carefully, trying to imagine what would interest 18-year-old boys in our hospital and work. We decided they should choose, after hearing a brief account of what we did. The great concern of the mission authorities was that the national and international press would disrupt this private visit. We could trust our local people but expected interference from local government officials nearby, who we heard were being offered bribes to help with transport. When the great day came, we actually blocked the mission landing strip to all incoming aircraft except for the Geelong party's flight. It was done by rolling 44-gallon drums down and across the runway. It was effective, and the Prince's party arrived, only to be set to work at once to roll the drums away and up the hill.

The boys were accommodated in the main mission house, in dormitories and large rooms, which had been cleaned and de-bugged specially. The washing facilities (bucket showers) and the loos (pit latrines) were out the back and shared by the whole party as well as staff.

I remember the first breakfast together. We were under instructions to treat all the boys equally and integrate them as much as possible into our mission life, including mealtimes. I was sitting at a long table eating my cereal and fruit, when I found a boy hovering over the empty chair next to me. A gentle voice said hesitatingly, 'Can I sit here?' My affirmative was at once acknowledged and I found the Prince next to me and asking eager questions. I quickly established that he was interested in our hospital, but focused on the strange tropical diseases he had heard so much about. We talked about TB and malaria and I offered to explain more in the hospital.

The programme was soon worked out, and started with a full tour of all parts of the institutions: primary school; teacher training college; theological college; girls' high school; hospital; boats, jetty and villages. I had to give a brief talk about health and how they could cope with local conditions, heat and insects; what to eat and drink and what not to; how to prevent mosquito bites becoming infected; and to avoid snakes and poisonous spiders. I think I put them off thoroughly! I had to spell it out as I knew they planned to climb the local high hill, called Mount Patsi-patsi, next morning and I often had to deal with the problems of expats. The Prince acknowledged that he had been kitted out in some of his grandfather's tropical gear – shorts and long socks with holes in the back, as well as his plimsolls. Naturally the Aussie boys were more appropriately dressed. I was worried and watched anxiously for their return that evening. Next morning I was called to see Prince Charles and several other boys, suffering from sunburn and blisters. Charles'e blisters were horrendous; he had a huge one on his heel and sole, caused by walking in extreme heat in hot, ill-fitting rubber shoes. Of course, he was stoical. I lanced the blister, disinfected and bound it all up impressively and put him in flip-flops which allowed him to walk without much pain. He recovered and I was proud that I had been of service to him.

He came back to the hospital later to hear all about malaria in particular. I had my laboratory technician, Barbara, set up slides for him to see and he spent an afternoon poring through the microscopes at the stained parasites. He was truly interested. We thought highly of him and his friends.

The local village people could not tell who was who in the party, so the Prince was well hidden in the crowd of young white men. An amusing story was told of how he and a group of boys were running on a village path when an old woman in a grass skirt popped up, holding an artefact in upstretched hands to several boys. Prince Charles thought it was a present for him, but the woman said severely to him, 'I want money, and then you can have it.' He was not carrying any, so left it behind.

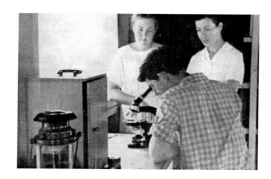

*Prince Charles with me and Barbara Axten at St Barnabas Hospital,
where he showed a keen interest in microscopic slides...*

I observed him several times walking around our large debba-debba (garden square), looking rather lost and not knowing where to go or what to do. When I asked him, he said he could not believe he had no one following him and could walk out on his own. He loved it.

On their last night there was a huge feast in a local village, about three miles' walk away, across a wide river. We usually waded across, but for some reason the mission tractor was ordered and we all sat on the trailer to be bumped along the tracks and over the river. It was an amazing evening with speeches, singing and dancing, and eating (roast pig). I kept a weather eye on my royal charge, especially what he ate; but all was well. I found him making for home on foot and in the midst of a large group of local young men and women, continuing their good time. Some boys were attacking the ripe sugar cane and teaching the visiting team how to break it, strip it with their teeth and eat it – delicious. I half expected to be called to repair royal teeth next morning but was not needed.

\*\*\*

But back to our routine. Were the patrols of value? And how did they help the people? I invested a lot of time – days and weeks – in visiting many difficult and remote villages. I spent hours and days walking and climbing mountains. It was challenging. We slept usually in a village rest house: a wood and bamboo house with a palm roof. We each had a mat and a mosquito net; it was very public and we were objects of great curiosity.

Early on, Lancelot, my medical assistant, came to me laughing and said, 'Dr Pene – the people are asking me if you are a man or a woman!' As I was young and had long blonde hair, I found this very amusing. I learned to help the people by insisting on bathing in the rivers with the women. They loved to bathe with me and made sure I was just like them. Especially they played with my hair – never having come across straight hair before. The alternative to the river was a bucket shower (which I have already mentioned). It meant cold water, in a screened-off corner with slatted floor – usually with crowds of children underneath the house, waiting hopefully for us to drop the soap. We usually did! If you wonder about his name, Lancelot was probably called after a missionary. He was a Papuan who had been mission-educated, and later he named his daughter after me.

Luggage was a big issue. Everything we took had to be carried by porters, whom we paid by trading tobacco or salt or some other popular commodity. We had one rucksack each for our personal belongings – clothes, towel and net. Then we were allowed a food sack – just one can of either meat or fish per day to share among us. How I disliked the tinned fish! This was the only meagre concession the mission allowed, deviating from the policy that we should only eat what each village gave us in payment for the medicines, vaccines, etc. we gave them. The villagers were very poor and their basic diet was sweet potato, yam and sometimes, but rarely, pork or fish. So our food depended on the season of the year and the harvest. If the harvest was good, then we ate well – as many sweet potato or yam as we could eat; I did not find this easy for breakfast, but I learned the hard way.

One morning, I was being pulled up the mountain by Lancelot and I was really struggling to keep going. He said to me, 'Pene – how many potatoes did you eat for breakfast today?' I replied, 'Two, I think.' As I sat at the top, he then lectured me: 'You need to eat more.' (Not many people have ever said that to me.) He said, 'If you want to climb these mountains you must eat a whole plate of yams or potatoes for breakfast to give you enough energy.' I think I weakly said, 'But I don't like them for breakfast.' 'You must force yourself – look how much I have helped you today.' He was quite right of course and I tried hard to do as he said. All this yam and potato depended on the villagers having a good stock for themselves. If they were hungry, then so were we. I recall one patrol when the villagers sent us a message to say they had little food and we should bring rations with us.

This meant adding a sack of rice to our load. Rice for three weeks (with nothing added) is pretty awful. On the last weekend of that patrol we were all protein-starved. We arrived at one village where the mission teacher welcomed us to his house. There were chickens running around outside and we looked longingly at them. The teacher's wife took the hint and put one in the pot for our dinner. It was tough – but no matter – it went very quickly and we all felt better. I think the discipline of those weeks out in the villages stood me in good stead in the years to come when I was working to help very poor people in refugee camps.

## Accidents and near misses

When people ask me, 'Were you in danger or frightened at any time?', I tend to laugh it off, but there were some moments when I thought I might have 'reached my end' though it wasn't so and I was always kept safe to continue. I was most scared in the St Gabriel, when the mountains seemed too near or when on one occasion the single engine stuttered and very nearly stopped. The pilots were marvellous and gave me confidence on the whole, except for one who delighted in surfing along the edge of the sea or chasing dogs down grass airstrips.

One time when I was patrolling in the Denoua Mountains, the rains came down heavily and the rivers rose alarmingly. We had to cross the big river without the benefit of even a cane bridge. The river had vast boulders of rock joining our path on each side. Our line started to cross, jumping from rock to rock. I hung back, very scared. My walking partner was Father Brian, a very tall man with long arms. He went ahead of me, saying, 'Just hang on to my hand and I will pull you across.' It worked until we were halfway across. Then there were two boulders with fast and deep water in between and it was impossible to stretch across. Only a long jump would get anyone across the deep channel. Brian went first successfully, leaving me behind alone on a rock. I had to go forward in faith. Brian held out his long left arm and encouraged me – 'Come on, jump for my hand.' I froze and prayed. I could not reach his hand. Then he held out his little finger and I stretched further, finally hooking my right little finger around his and completing my jump with his help. It was terrifying.

Another water emergency came my way at a village called Sirisiri, many miles inland from Dogura. Our group was walking at midday – aiming to reach the village for dinner and sleep. The village were expecting us – luckily, as it turned out. Unwisely, we sat down for lunch in a dry river bed. There was a storm brewing in the hills around us with thunder and lightning. It was not raining where we were so we took no notice until our medical orderly suddenly shouted, 'Look – water – run!!' Coming towards us very fast was a wall of water headed by a great wave. We ran – abandoning our packs – each to the nearest bank. I reached the bank just as the wave reached us and clung onto the tree roots. The power of that water was overwhelming and I have never forgotten it or sat down in a dry river bed again. Then it started to rain. It poured with sheets of water, drenching us to our skins – as though we weren't already that wet. It was cold too – even there in the tropics. Luckily for me, some of our men had run to my bank and they came to pull me out of the now fast-flowing river. At least half our group had run to the opposite bank, which was on the village side – so we were hopeful they would give the alarm and villagers would come to rescue us. We had no food or clean water. The men decided to build a shelter from brushwood and trees, but that rain came through everything and we remained wet through.

The darkness came early that night and we could do nothing except pray and sing. We were confident we would be found. And we were – after a few hours we saw lights twinkling from lamps on the far bank and we made out figures of men running up and down the river bank. I watched fascinated while they stripped tree bark to form a long rope, which they attached around one young man's waist. He then attacked the river, and after a few false starts, when he was hauled back to his side, he crossed successfully and we pulled him out on our side – joy, oh joy! He attached the rope end to a sturdy tree trunk and invited us to cross the river holding the rope bridge. By now more men had come across to help us. Our party began the journey across and I knew I had to face it. My young trainee nurse was as terrified as me. The men picked her up and fixed her hands to the rope and held them there, proceeding to cross safely – almost carrying her. Then it was my turn to be picked up and attached to the tree rope. Now I was in that raging river again and it was hard to hold on. I was pulled down all the time. My escort held my hands firmly on the rope and made me move along it. My problem was to keep my head above water. My escort, bless him, was so intent on holding onto my hands and keeping them on the rope that he sat on my head. I struggled to push him off my head. I survived and reached the far bank – much to the relief of my medical assistant, waiting for me and watching. We dried off in the village, conducted the clinic next day and went on our way very sobered.

***

On another patrol in the Daga Mountains, I was walking (climbing) with several priests on a combined patrol (medical and evangelistic). The walk was long and hard and I suppose I drank some bad water. I became ill and when we stopped for the night in a small village, I knew I could not go on. I had a bad attack of dysentery. I was invited to sleep in a small rest house – the usual grass house on high stilts, reached by a notched tree trunk – not ideal for someone with my complaint. The rest of the group went on that night to the next place where they were due at services next morning. I felt lonely and ill. I got worse. Only a scared young trainee nurse was with me to look after me. She was frightened too. Lying on my mat on the bamboo floor, I was aware of talking in the next room. It sounded serious. I asked the nurse what was going on. After a bit she came back and, hesitating, said, 'It is a meeting of chiefs and they are discussing what to do with your body when you die.' This was my challenge and I determined not to bother them like this. I got better and, though very weak, I went back next day down to the coast, where we hitched a lift on a canoe back home. At least, I lost a lot of weight.

We quite often came across very ill people in their homes – both children and adults. Maternal health was a big problem. Women gave birth in their own homes and very often alone; they had to build themselves a small birthing house in the village, and I was later to discover the significance of this.

***

One formative experience for me was meeting a very ill woman, being carried on a home-made stretcher along the narrow path from her village towards Dogura. Her husband was leading the way and I recognised him as a 'big man' or chief, whom I had advised that he must bring his wife down to the hospital for her next birth. He had not, and she had almost ex-sanguinated during childbirth. I tried to save her but could not do so in that remote place. I challenged the man, saying, 'Why didn't you bring her? I told you she might die.' He nonchalantly replied, 'I had to harvest my coffee and could not bring her. It is easy to get another wife, but not another harvest.' I was dumbfounded, but this reply changed my career plans as I vowed to fight for women's health and rights.


## My Brother John, 1968

Totally unexpectedly for me, one day in late 1967, I had a letter from my brother John (a young vicar now), telling me he had applied to be rector of a church in Port Moresby. He proposed to join me in PNG with his wife and family. I was thrilled. What a difference it would make to me to have family close by to visit.

It took several months for John and family to sort out the job and housing and to be accepted by the church, where there had never been a family man before. The family now included Ben, aged two years, but there was a second on the way. What an effort it must have been for my sister-in-law, Loveday, to leave her family and the safety of the British medical services to live and work in a foreign tropical country. Certainly they both stepped out in faith. I managed to get a few days off to fly over the mountains to Port Moresby to meet them in January 1968 and settle them into their new rectory in Boroko, a new suburb of Port Moresby. It was just wonderful to see them all. I was only with them a few days before I had to return to Dogura, but not before arranging for them to visit me. Next was the excitement of the birth of their daughter, Jane, who chose to make her entry on the same day as my youngest brother Rob's wedding day in Scotland. In fact, Jane's arrival was announced at the wedding reception, where we sent a telegram saying, 'Love from John, Loveday, Pene, Ben and – Jane too.' What a way to hear of your first granddaughter's birth so far away! Loveday did not have an easy time in hospital or after going home. I think the heat was just too much for her. But Jane thrived and I was able to be with them a few days. I loved looking after my little nephew, Ben, a dear little boy who insisted on sleeping on the floor, not a bed. I think it was cooler.

In their second year at Boroko, John became ill with hepatitis. It was a common illness there, contracted by many foreigners. John turned yellow and was so ill that he was admitted to hospital. The jaundice increased daily and he could not eat anything. We became more and more worried as the doctors started to shake their heads and say there was nothing more they could do. I knew that a few foreigners did die every year from hepatitis. Loveday was desperate but strong. After about four weeks, the jaundice came down just a little and then they said he could go home, but he should go away from here to convalesce in a cooler place. We had almost no money between us so I sent an SOS to our good relations in Australia, asking if anyone could take us all in. I would go with them to help with the children. The response was immediate and positive. Cousins Ann and Alastair Robson would lend us their cottage in Palm Beach, Sydney, for as long as needed. It was heaven-sent. Off we all went, in November 1969. And it worked. John gradually recovered and Loveday and the children had a good holiday. After one month, I left for my home leave and could take reassuring news of John to my anxious parents.

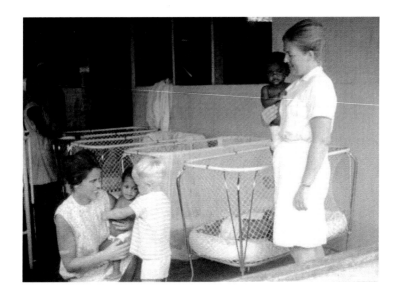

*With Loveday and Ben on their first visit to Dogura – I am holding an orphan baby*

John did return to Boroko for a year, leaving in June 1971, but then he joined World Vision and worked in a lot of poor countries, including Bangladesh and India, then at base in USA. Finally, he and Loveday decided to emigrate to Australia with their younger children and they built a house in north Sydney.

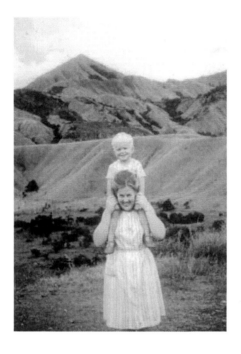

*With Ben*

## Home Leave

In January 1970, leaving Sydney, I went on home leave for four months (one month for each year served) to learn more about treating diseases of women. By this time, my parents had retired to Stover, and I did not know my brothers and their wives and children well, if at all, especially the youngest, Robert, who was by now at university and had just married Sue... There were always new things about my family to learn when I came back!

I had no money, so had to find a job. I managed to secure a Senior House Officer (SHO) appointment at the famous Queen Charlotte's Hospital in west London. I don't know why they gave me the job – probably they were curious to have someone who had worked in a remote place. Curiosity did not last long. I had a lot of difficulty adjusting to British healthcare and expectations. My immediate supervisor – the registrar – soon decided that his responsibility was to protect the patients from me. I tended to make a diagnosis and start treatment before asking someone what to do. This was not right in their eyes; SHOs were not supposed to know anything and always to refer their patients upwards for decisions. I must have been a great trial – especially when I often told them that I had seen lots of such cases and knew how to treat it. The crunch came for me the day that I treated an emergency condition in the labour ward without calling my registrar. It was a condition (inverted uterus) I had seen regularly at Dogura but it was very rare in the UK. It transpired that my registrar had never seen a case, so he was really offended and very angry with me for not calling him immediately, despite the patient making a good recovery. Also, I was not good with private patients, whom we were expected to look after for our consultants, attending to their day-to-day or night problems. My tendency was to stand no nonsense from them and when a weathy society mother-to-be sent for me in the night because she could not sleep, I told her to shut up and not be stupid – or the equivalent. I was never again allowed to see her and was given a right rocket by the consultant – but he was pocketing her money, not me. However, I learned a lot in the six months and was lucky to be given a three-month follow-up studentship at the partner hospital – Chelsea Hospital for Women – where I brushed up my gynaecology and anaesthetics.

Then I had to make another big decision – what would I do next? I had been offered a job with the PNG/Australian Government but I was being advised by professional colleagues to continue my education at home and take my master's degree in obstetrics and gynaecology. It was a hard choice but I loved the overseas work and could not bear the limitations of the UK NHS. My parents badly wanted me to stay at home and work nearby, but they never stood in my way, encouraging me instead to follow my dreams and calling.

\*\*\*

I had to pay my own way back across the world. It was the time of the £10 emigration ticket to Australia so I decided to try for it. I succeeded and flew off to Brisbane and Port Moresby at the expense of the Australian Government. They of course still administered PNG – providing most of the funds for services and all the administration. I turned up one November day in Port Moresby and went to the Ministry of Health and offered myself for a suitable job. They were expecting me and had lined up a job to offer me. I was surprised and overawed to be offered the post of Medical Superintendent of Mount Hagen District Hospital in the Highlands – to start immediately. I had no experience or qualifications in hospital management, other than what I had picked up in the mission hospitals. I suppose someone in the Ministry had made some enquiries!

# Chapter 3: PNG Again – A new post in the Highlands

## Mount Hagen

I had never been to Mount Hagen and was apprehensive about taking over as leader and manager of a new place where I knew no one. I was only 31 years old and the senior surgeon was a highly qualified Australian man of more than 60. The Australian matron, Jill Kennedy, soon became a good friend and she schooled me well in running a hospital. The hospital was very basic, though it was the district referral hospital for a huge population of several million. We saw everything – a lot of trauma from tribal fights and road accidents, and many maternity cases – mostly complications of delivery – and we lost too many women. Here I began to do the anaesthetics as there was no one else – and of course I did the maternity. Paediatrics also became my charge. We always had wards full of very sick children: none had been immunised so we saw measles, whooping cough and even diphtheria. I settled into the hospital routine – no chance of patrols here, as the hospital was too busy to be left. Nor was there any time off, so I quickly became very tired. I had my own house – a nice one near the hospital, where I was too often disturbed by women keening as they grieved loudly over the loss of a child or loved one.

## Jimmi River

One of the Anglican mission stations was in my catchment area – Jimmi River, five minutes' flying over the mountains. Peter and Olive Robin came in regularly to Mount Hagen and they were a good support to me at that time. Olive, a nurse, was investigating the illness of a lot of children in the villages around Jimmi. The children showed cerebral retardation at nine months and over; they failed to develop and could not walk or talk. I tried to help and the mission found a wonderful British physiotherapist, Liz Roberts, to go to Jimmi and help the children. After a while, a visiting paediatrician came up with the answer. The children were iodine deficient – we found a lot of goitres among the women. So we started a big programme of iodine supplementation for all the babies and toddlers. Things improved for the families – and Liz and I have maintained our friendship over the years since.

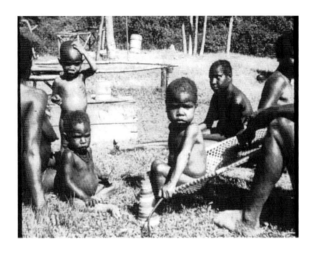

*Iodine deficient children, Jimmi River*

## Whooping Cough Epidemic

Then came one of the busiest and most taxing times of my life so far. There was an outbreak of pertussis (whooping cough) in the totally unimmunised child population. It swept through villages locally and far afield. Many died of asphyxia from blockage of their airways. Our hospital was overflowing. The paediatrician from Goroka, Jim Bidduph, came over to help me and show me what to do for the children. It was mostly a question of unblocking the airways by tipping them head-down and sucking out the mucus. This is really the remit of a physiotherapist which we did not have, so I sent for Liz Roberts from Jimmi mission. She came and stayed with me for six months – she was a marvellous help and saved many young lives. I will never forget those little babies who could not fight and who we lost. I hope that no governments will stop immunising against pertussis. We did

79

follow up the epidemic with a massive immunisation campaign throughout the Highlands, but it was too late for many.


## Port Moresby Interlude

Soon after this I was recalled to Port Moresby for about nine months, to help out in the absence of their obstetrics consultant on leave. Actually, I worked as a registrar, which suited my limited skills more. I did not much enjoy this episode of my career: it was far removed from the remote work I loved. I was back to treating expatriates and educated locals, but I also began teaching medical students, which I did enjoy. During this time I managed to pick up a severe attack of pneumonia, which took me some time to get over. Then the Ministry of Health gave me a choice: stay in Moresby maternity unit or go to Chimbu Hospital in the Highlands as medical superintendent.


## Kundiawa (Chimbu), 1972-73

The Chimbu tribe are renowned for their fighting spirit, large numbers and especially their tradition of pay-back killing. For me there was no choice and accordingly I set off again for another new place in the mountains. Chimbu Hospital was a real bush hospital again, set in a valley between massive mountains. Arriving by air was terrifying – the plane had to curve around very close to Mount Michael (a massive 12,000 feet) and drop down into a narrow valley and, two right angles later, line up with the grass landing strip and bump down. We had just one fatal crash while I was there. A young Australian pilot was practising his landing with an instructor, as they all had to do on the more remote airstrips. He made twenty attempts to land but had to abort each time. On the twenty-first attempt, he crashed the plane – fatally for himself and his instructor.

The hospital wards were made of bush straw roofs on a concrete base with walls of plaited grass leaves. There was quite a good operating theatre, heavily used, because it was the referral hospital for many thousands of violent Chimbu people. It had around 200 beds, but we admitted anyone needing care, so could have any number of extra people sleeping on mats in the wards.

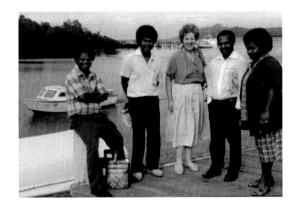

*With some of my medical students at Port Moresby*

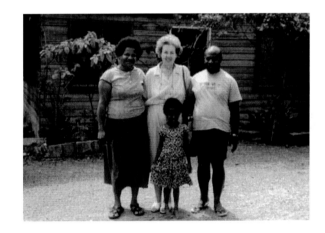

*With a Papuan priest, Caedman, and his family*

## Our Staff

There were two young English doctors there before me, Andy and David. They had come out as British VSOs. Neither had much experience but their huge enthusiasm made up for their lack of experience. Again, I took the women patients and the children, while they looked after most others. We were quickly introduced to the horrible trauma of arrow wounds. The

Chimbu arrows had a wicked barb and couldn't be pulled out. Sometimes we had to push an arrow through an arm or leg and cut it behind the barb to get it out – pretty horrible. My worst case was a young medical orderly who was called to treat some wounded fighters. He got in the way of an arrow, which pierced his eye. This presented a dilemma to us. If we left it in, infection was inevitable. If we extracted it there would be no way to stop the bleeding. After signs of infection began, we tried to extract it but were unsuccessful – sadly, the man died from the haemorrhage.

## The Tribal Chiefs

I was in despair over us spending so much time repairing needless trauma. It meant neglecting the many problems of the mothers and children. I know that one day I 'snapped' when I was unable to perform an emergency Caesarean section because the operating theatre was occupied by an injured man. Men always came first in that place. I spoke to many Chimbu chiefs about this problem, but they simply did not understand why it was a problem to me; it was not to them – there were plenty more women available. Tribal fights usually came at certain seasons, so we could anticipate them, but so could the chiefs. In my second year I took the initiative of talking to the area chiefs. I was quite tough with them. I said, 'If you are going to fight this year, please plan to charter planes for the wounded men to go to Goroka for treatment, because our/your hospital is full and we cannot help your men.' They meekly agreed and did send a planeload to the Goroka referral hospital. At Christmas that year, the chiefs approached me and asked for a doctor to be present at their fight to give emergency treatment. Amused, I asked the two young doctors for a volunteer. Andy jumped at it and got his camera ready. He was three days at the fight and had wonderful stories and pictures. Apparently it was all a bit of a show. The men were all lined up facing each other until the chiefs said 'Go'. They had lunch breaks, during which bows and arrows were laid down, but not until all had had their picture taken by a willing Andy. He thought it was all very friendly and very few were wounded those days.

One day a paramount chief lay dying in the hospital. His heart was failing. Andy asked me to see him, as I was considered to be old and wise and I had a responsibility to treat the old man. After I had examined him and was solemnly telling his relatives that we could not cure him, the old man spoke urgently into my ear, saying, 'You must not let me die yet. I have not told my heirs where I have buried my money.' Luckily I was aware of this custom. The coffee growers all stashed their large amounts of cash at the foot of an ancient tree or some other secret place. The secret was passed on to the chosen son or tribal heir before death. But the heir had not arrived and time was fast running out for the old chief. Of course, the tribesmen were equally worried as the tribe needed that money. There was a happy outcome when his son, also an old man, turned up just in time, after which the old chief died peacefully.

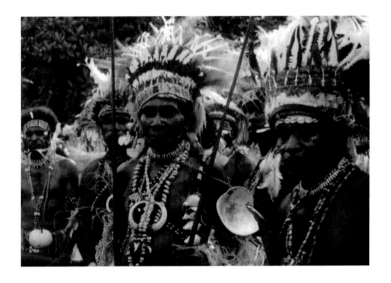

*Tribal chiefs*

Lots of young men did not die peacefully. Rather, they met a violent end through pay-back killing between two tribes. I first came up against this in the hospital. Almost all the male medical orderlies were from the same nearby tribe. One day I couldn't find any medical orderlies. I was told that they had locked themselves into the operating theatre (the only solid building), keeping out of sight of any one looking for them for a killing. A man in their rival clan had been killed last night and his friends were out to find a young man from the killer's tribe to pay back. The young men were terrified and I had to promise them I would not give them away, though eventually I had to turn them out of the theatre to do an operation.


## Culture Clashes

Another local custom that caused us lots of problems concerned transport for pregnant women. It took me some time to find out why it was so difficult for women to arrange transport from their village to the hospital when having a complication in childbirth. I knew that the women built themselves a 'birthing hut' on their land, and went away from their family into this for the birth. They remained in that hut until all bleeding had stopped and then they set light to and burned the hut, always with any bedding or clothes that had had contact with blood or other fluids. I was told that a woman's blood during or after childbirth was totally defiling and anything coming into contact with it must be burned. This extended to any vehicle or stretcher used for a woman seeking help. A man was bound to burn his vehicle if it had carried a defiling woman. So the price of a post-partum referral was the cost of a new truck! It really did happen. Consequently, my efforts to encourage early referral of women with post-partum haemorrhage had little or no chance of success without overcoming the superstition of the people and their tradition of 'evil spirits'.

Killings were an everyday event, and I soon found out from the Australian Chief of Police that Australian law demanded that a qualified doctor should do a post mortem examination on any violent death. This was an extraordinary transfer of law to be applied across the cultures: it was totally contrary to Chimbu custom and spelt big trouble for the doctor assigned. The task usually fell to me as I was the only one with the training and experience. I used to feel very vulnerable when there were 1,000 or more angry tribesmen surrounding the bush mortuary, waiting to take the desecrated body home, which they did as soon as I had finished. Mostly there was nothing complicated about determining the cause of death, which was generally major trauma such as an axe to the head or an arrow through the heart. I tried hard to get the policeman to relax the rule but he would not. All he offered me was a police escort at the hospital mortuary for post mortems on young men. I just could not see the point of the dangerous exercise and I was ready to take on Canberra itself on the matter, rather than expose my staff. In the end it came to just that – and I won, though it led to my departure from PNG. It happened like this.

## The last straw for me

At Christmas 1972, a young man was brought in by the police, killed in a road accident nearby, with a massive head injury. Everyone could see what had happened. I suggested to the police chief that he did not need a post mortem as the cause of death was not suspicious. He still insisted I go ahead, so I did. After my morning rounds the next day, I walked out to the mortuary, expecting the usual mass of angry men – but there were only women there, keening and rolling around on the ground as usual. Because of the absence of men, the police chief had sent only one old policeman as escort, whereas there were usually twenty or so.

I thought the quiet was a bit strange but was not prepared for what happened next. As soon as I went to open the mortuary door, several tribeswomen leapt up at me. They seized me, shouting loudly for all the other women to join them, attacking me. I called in vain to the policeman, who did nothing but stand and watch. I was a bit bruised and battered but not seriously hurt: it was more my spirit that was wounded and I was angry that the policeman had not stopped them. When I challenged the old man, he said in his best Pidgin, 'Em fight olgether bilong Meri – nogat bilong man.' In English that means, 'This is women's business not men's; it has nothing to do with me, a man.' That made me even more cross and I challenged the police chief who just laughed and said, 'Well, you are all right, so why should we lock up the women who did this?' As I was really in sympathy with the women and thought the whole business stupid, I did not pursue it with the local people. Instead I sent off a cable (there was no email or fax there then) to the Ministry of Heath telling them what had happened and recommending the practice of post mortems be rescinded in Chimbu. I copied it to the Health Department in Canberra, and finally got a positive response. They agreed with me and said that in these sorts of exceptional situations the law need not be applied – at the discretion of the local police chief. *That* was the sting in the tail, but he was replaced very soon afterwards.

I was very upset emotionally after this episode, so I took some leave due to me and travelled back to Papua to visit old friends. I started to think very hard about my future. Did I really want to spend all my professional life in PNG? Should I move on?

## My Departure

Independence was just around the corner and things did not appear very calm on the ground. Port Moresby was becoming a violent city, and even the rural areas were experiencing violent hold-ups from gangs of youths. I was helped a lot by my mission friends to come to a decision, and before I returned to Chimbu I gave in my notice to the Health Ministry. I think they were expecting it and I think they were not that sorry; I had always been a bit of a thorn in the flesh and I was very demanding of them. For instance, in my first year there I exposed the hidden facts about gender discrimination between male and female doctors. I was being paid roughly one third as much as my male counterparts for the same job. I won this one too, but it did not make me popular with the civil servants or the politicians. I was convinced that there was another job waiting for me; I just had to discover what it was. As before, I decided to take a break at home to consider.

## My next move

I duly flew home, having enticed my stay-at-home father to venture to Switzerland with Mother (who was not a stay-at-home) to meet me and have a holiday. My parents, who were getting older, had retired and as I have said, they were now living at Stover – in their dream house which I, too, loved.

Father was excited by the idea of Switzerland for a holiday and meeting place. Those were the days of Motorail and he booked their tickets on the train cross-country to Berne. Clearly, they greatly enjoyed their journey, later telling me excitedly about sitting in station cafés and having croissants and coffee for breakfast. Meanwhile, I booked my flight to Athens, where I knew someone who had a small flat in the town centre, which she let me stay in for a week to see the city. I had a good time – all to myself. Then I got on the train and went first through Italy to France and thence by train to Berne to join my parents. They were there to meet me at the station. I could not believe that they had made it there with the car, but they had, and we had a wonderful ten days, first in a hotel on a lakeside, then, best of all, in a small family hotel in a village called Wilderswil near Interlaken. We took the mountain railway to the Schynige Platt to see the wild flowers and even went up over the Jungfrau; and we got to know each other again, having lots to say. Then we drove home.

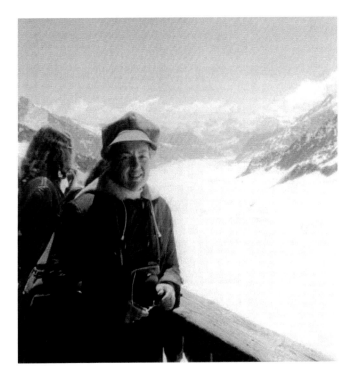

*On holiday in Switzerland, 1973*

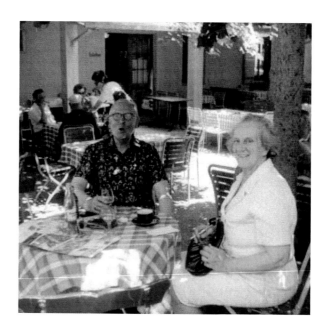

*Mother and Dad in Switzerland*

Father had not had enough and decided another trip, this time to Scotland, would be in order. I was delighted and off we went – my mother, father and me. I remember it as a lovely time. I learned from Tim, then working as a factor in the Highlands, how to stalk – I was fit enough now. Dad and I fished together and talked a lot. I was waiting for my next call and they knew that. As always, they supported me and my decisions, though they really wanted me at home: our beloved Vi had recently died of cancer and my parents had no one to look after them.

## A Call

One day when I was up a mountain, a telephone call from Australia came for me in the hotel. Dad did not know who it was – someone called Graham – but agreed to get me to ring him back. With beating heart, I rang the overseas number in Melbourne. Graham was a friend of my brother John and Director of World Vision Australia (a Christian NGO). His message was short and breathtaking: 'Pene, will you lead a medical team into Cambodia now, at once, to care for all the people displaced by war in Phnom Penh, the capital city? We have one other doctor and two nurses waiting to go, but we need you.' The call had come and I knew what my answer was to be at once. After a brief discussion with my parents, I rang back and said, 'Yes – when do you want me?' Graham said, 'How about next week? The need is urgent. I will book you a flight to Melbourne next week and will orientate you for two days before sending you off to Cambodia.' My parents were wonderful, as ever, and started to help me get ready.

I did a lot of research into Cambodia and the war situation there. I re-packed my bags with tropical gear – Cambodia was to be hot, but I was travelling economy class and could not take much with me. I needed some medical gear. Then, goodbyes all round again and off I flew into the unknown once more.

Reflecting on my snap decision, which influenced my future life, I know now that it was God's plan for me to go to Cambodia, because I was needed there and could make a difference to some people. At the time, I had just 'gone with the flow' and taken each day as it came, trying to cram in my goodbyes again to brothers and parents – doubly hard to say goodbye to my brothers' little children, whom I already loved dearly. My brothers never criticised me for going off again, but I knew in my heart that there was good reason for them to think I was needed at home now. Dad was sure I was right and helped me in every way. Mum was supportive too, though she did not want me to go at all. It was a huge step for me and I felt unprepared for the new challenge.

# Chapter 4: Cambodia I: 1973-75

In Melbourne 48 hours later, and very tired, I was introduced to World Vision Australia (WVA). My brother John had worked for some time for World Vision International (WVI) out of USA, so I knew a good deal about them already. I enjoyed meeting the two newly-recruited nurses, Margaret and Joan, both of them experienced overseas. Indeed, I had known Margaret in PNG, so we were able to help each other. Margaret stayed with me right to the end of my time in Cambodia. She was an excellent public health nurse, much loved by all her patients. Dr Jim Sinclair was the fourth team member. He was a retired doctor from Melbourne and it was because of him that we were going to Cambodia. He had already been there to scout for what we should be doing. He had convinced the Cambodian church, whose guest he was, that they should approach World Vision to send in a medical relief team, so he had a plan in mind for us.

In September 1973 our small team flew into Phnom Penh, the capital city of Cambodia. My very first reaction to my phone call in Scotland had been, 'Where is Cambodia?' Now I still have to ask people if they have ever heard about Kampuchea. Their response is generally no. And, 'Have you ever seen Angkor Wat?' 'No.' 'Have you ever heard about the killing fields?' Silence follows. As I discover again and again, Cambodia is not well known in England or even anywhere outside East Asia. Australians are better informed – but Cambodia is not so far away from them.

Cambodia, in South East Asia, was once known not as 'The Killing Fields', but as 'The Land of Paradise'. Most of the Khmer, or Kampuchean, people (Cambodians) had led a peaceful, harmonious existence cultivating rice in the countryside. In the past fifty years, however, Cambodia has been turned upside-down. I have found the BBC website helpful when remembering the sequence of events – particularly News Online's guide to its turbulent history since 1953.

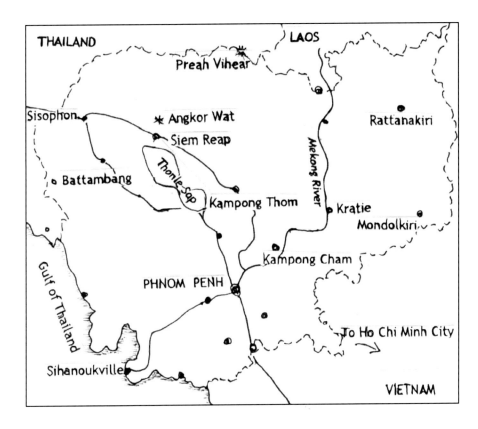

*Location map –* **CAMBODIA**

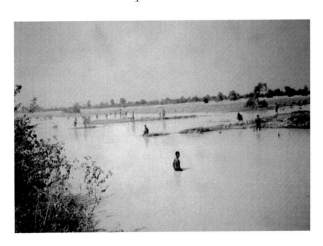

*This is Cambodia*

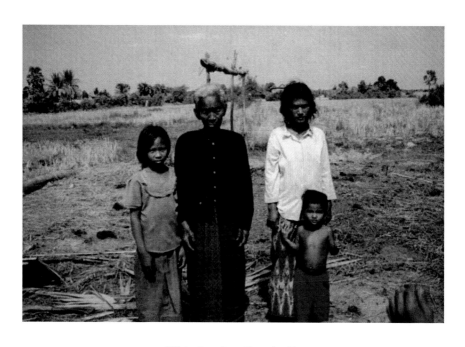

*This is also Cambodia*

In 1941, Prince Norodom Sihanouk became king, and managed to bring the country to full independence from the French by 1953. One year after that, he relinquished his throne to his father, and entered the political arena. Later, he became the prime minister and head of state. During this period he was keen to keep Cambodia out of the war being fought in neighbouring countries. He seemed reasonably successful in dealing with the external political pressure, but he failed to manage internal politics. Internally, he was opposed by both the leftist Khmer Rouge (Red Khmer or Khmer Communists) led by the infamous Pol Pot, and by the rightists (his own government). In early 1970, the king was overthrown and the monarchy abolished. A Khmer republic was established, led by General Lon Nol and supported by the Americans. Sihanouk went to China, where he decided to ally himself with his former enemy, the Khmer Rouge, to try to regain control of Cambodia. He became the head of state for the Khmer Rouge, but he had no actual power over Pol Pot or the Khmer Rouge soldiers. Between 1970 and 1975 civil war raged throughout Cambodia. The country was gradually engulfed by the Khmer Rouge soldiers, and the government of the new republic grew totally corrupt. Society became chaotic. Many who hated corruption were psychologically coerced into joining the Khmer Rouge to fight the government of the republic.

In April 1975, the Khmer Rouge captured the whole country. Soon after the Khmer Rouge took over, they turned Cambodia into the 'Land of Killing Fields'. Much has been written about this and a famous film made. People were evacuated from the cities to work in the countryside. Life under the Khmer Rouge's merciless regime became meaningless and worthless. My Khmer medical team, along with their families, were among the many innocent people forced to do hard labour with little food to eat. In 1977, my dear friend Thivan (my interpreter) was executed by the Khmer Rouge. Kem Kanyaket, her dear friend and another of our team's interpreters, survived the killing. Her story comes later. During the reign of the Khmer Rouge, it is estimated that two million Cambodian people were killed. It was because fields full of human skulls were found outside Phnom Penh – where all the people who died in the torture prison had been buried – that the new name, 'the killing fields', was given.

In early 1979 Cambodia came under another regime, this one supported by the Vietnamese Government. For the ordinary people, worn out by hunger, torture and illness, this was liberation and the day (7th January) is still celebrated as 'Liberation Day'. The new regime was still communist and there was almost no money to address the awful situation in the country, especially the loss of all the educated people. But all that came later – a lot happened in between.

On a personal level, my time in Cambodia until I left in April 1975, when the Khmer Rouge conquered the city of Phnom Penh, was totally life-changing for me. Having begun by doing clinical medical work for the thousands who needed us, I realised very soon that my previous choice of public health – the health of the many, rather than treatment of the individual – was the way for me. My life at this time involved a series of difficult choices.

## Our start

We (the Australian medical team) were greeted in 1973 at Phnom Penh airport by Carl Harris (just appointed Director of the World Vision

93

Cambodia programme), along with Minh Voan (the Cambodian Deputy Director) and other Cambodian staff of the new office. They had rented a house for us in a central part of Phnom Penh; No 10 Keo Chea was my first, but not last, home in Cambodia.

## Setting up house

It was a French-style villa like many in the city, with thick walls which gave useful protection, large rooms and high ceilings. There were two storeys, with a flat roof on which you could sit or stand – or hang out washing. We had beds but no mattresses, so our first task before going to bed that night was to go out to the shops and purchase mattresses or foam rubber to make do. That was an adventure in itself for which we needed a guide/interpreter. We had a Khmer cook as well. He did all the food shopping and produced three meals a day – all Cambodian food, of course. We soon learned to appreciate the rice-based fish and vegetable diet, though at first we often succumbed to the French bread baguettes sold on every corner. The house soon became a real home and safe haven for us all. Our Cambodian staff were based here and our plans were made from here. We adapted an outbuilding – a sort of larder – to be our medical and drug store.

Carl Harris was an American minister with previous experience of working in developing countries, but none of conflict or war situations. He was a 'no-nonsense' boss, who expected obedience from all of us – especially us women – and this did not augur well for me, used as I was to being the boss myself. However, he had plenty of imagination and a firm wish to provide massive relief for all the displaced people thronging the city. Our relationship improved as we each drew up our plans for making a difference there. I was given a lot of leeway to develop the medical relief programme, though money was scarce.

## Starting a clinic

Jim (Dr Jim Sinclair), our appointed leader, started by meeting the local church leaders and seeking their ideas for using our team. They had very little knowledge of health services, only knowing they were scarce and out of reach of most people, but they could also easily show us the many problems of the overcrowded city.

Even more important was the help we received from the Christian and Missionary Alliance medical staff. Dr Dean Kroh was an amazing, dedicated American doctor who was working with World Vision America to guide their project to build and establish a new children's hospital. With him were two nurses – Mary Lou and Barbara Neith – who readily took us to see their work in camp clinics they had set up. Both of them gradually became absorbed into our medical team, as Dr Kroh changed his way of working to concentrate on hospital development.

## Interpreters – the language

Having so soon encountered the language barrier, we knew that we could not talk to the people until we had interpreters, so our first task was to go and find English speakers wanting a job. On Dr Kroh's advice, we started at the only English-teaching high school in Phnom Penh, Beng Trabek. They told us that a number of girls had recently left school able to speak good English and, no doubt, looking for jobs. So we followed them up. We soon found Thivan, a very beautiful young Cambodian girl of nineteen years, who lived in the town centre, not far from our house. I was delighted to employ Thivan as my own dedicated translator. Dear Thivan became a great friend and like a sister to me. She told us such a lot about the culture and customs of Cambodia, as well as teaching me the Khmer language. Without Thivan and her young friends, the rest of my life and story might not have happened as it did. Thivan was so exhausted after a day working with me in the clinics that I employed a reserve translator, and Thivan brought along her close friend Kem Kanyaket (known as Kem or Kan), whom I know to this day as my adopted sister. The two of them spent hours and days helping us to go shopping, employ more staff and introduce ourselves to the medical authorities of the city and country.

## Touring the city

At that time Phnom Penh was a fortified city. There was barbed wire along all the streets and the riverbank. There were soldiers everywhere, ragged and shoeless but, above all, armed with grenades and shot guns. They wanted – and often needed – treatment, as much as many others. This presented a problem in our clinics, which were targeted at the poorest displaced people. The army had their own medical service as well as a hospital and we were very opposed to treating soldiers for their minor illnesses — more on this later – but our Cambodian staff were frightened of them and gave in easily, making me cross.

## Touring the hospitals

With Dr Jim, I started on visits to the hospitals of the city. I was truly shocked by what we found. After all, this had been a French colony and should surely have had a reasonable hospital service? The largest public hospital was called Preah Ket Malea. Situated in the centre of the city, it was indescribably awful – a vast concrete structure with a series of large, old-fashioned wards, no beds and neither water nor sanitation. The operating theatre was rudimentary, without essential equipment. There was usually no electricity, but that went for the rest of the city too – there might be four hours a day for a favoured location. The city water supply was running out, though I was glad to find Oxfam UK concentrating on renovating the supply, which was constantly sabotaged by the enemy.

There were two International Red Cross teams trying to start work in the hospitals. They had a very difficult task and were a huge standby to us when we needed to refer patients. There was a new children's hospital just starting, run by a young Swiss doctor, Beat Richner. He was an entertainer in his home country – and a famous cello player. Legend has it that he heard of the need in Cambodia and decided to raise money in Europe to take out there to help. He arrived in Phnom Penh with the proverbial 'suitcase full of dollars/francs', presented himself to the Ministry of Health and offered to build a children's hospital. Cambodians always say 'Yes', and who would say

'No' to an offer like this? The King was delighted and, politician that he was, he took personal credit for the new hospital, giving land near the city centre for the buildings. Beat became a good friend to us, and we referred many sick children to his expert care. He is still in Cambodia and still running children's hospitals around the country.

## Work Routine

Our team was not unanimous as to where and how to work. We wondered where we could make a difference in the face of the huge need. The church wanted us to set up clinics in their town centre base of Takhmau, south of the city. I felt that Takhmau was not where the largest number of displaced, homeless people was living and so I stuck out for a clinic in the city centre. No one thought that I would find a building to use – perhaps they did not know me. We found a huge group of displaced people camping out in a skeleton hotel, where there was not even a roof, but a basement and ground floor already constructed. People had moved in and made their homes in the basement, where there was some shelter and privacy. They constructed straw walls and wooden beds and had quite cosy homes – but again, with no sanitation or running water. With Thivan, I toured the camp in the hotel and talked to the leaders and people – mostly women. All had suffered hugely at the hands of the Khmer Rouge, who had systematically evacuated and destroyed their village homes in the countryside and driven all the survivors into Phnom Penh. The men were mostly killed or conscripted and never seen again. The women and children, with some old men, were starving and without money to buy food in the local markets. Many children were dying every day and there was no money to bury them.

At this time, I wrote the following passage in a diary. It has been slightly edited, but the situation was much as described then.

### Cambodiana Clinic 1973

*The unfinished Casino Cambodiana is a huge, impressive building, located on the banks of the Bassac River, with superb views across the Mekong River and, at the back, over the city of*

*Phnom Penh. It has seven floors of individual rooms, nearly 1,000 in all. The first floor is the reception area, with an impressive staircase leading up to a wide lobby, dining rooms, lounges and verandas. A pleasant swimming pool on a wide terrace, beside the river, completes the scene and conjures up the rich Western tourist who is meant to be lured to spend his vacation and his dollars, idling away days in the warm tropical sunshine.*

All this was only in dreams of a future which did not come to pass, for the hotel was not finished when the war broke out in 1970, and all work on it stopped, because there was no building material obtainable. In 1971, the government requisitioned the building shell as a transit camp for war refugees and it continued to be home to large numbers of displaced people till 1975, when Pol Pot had everyone thrown out.

In 1973, when I arrived there, there were 5,000 displaced Cambodians living there, though 'living' is hardly the right word. They were 'existing' in conditions that we from the developed world would find hard to imagine. They were not using the floors with bedrooms, with their individual rooms, bathrooms and balconies, for the owners had so far managed to contain the refugees on the first and ground floors. They had removed all staircases and blocked every access to the upper rooms.

*The refugees live a communal life in the corridors and spaces, with the only privacy created by hanging cloths or making straw screens around 'their' space. Imagine one hundred families living together in a hotel dining room. The basement or ground floor is popular. Two thousand people live among the foundations of this vast building. The floor is mud and often very wet. It is dark inside, which makes for more privacy and a feeling of 'homeliness'. Going down into this area reminds me of the dungeons of old castles at home, but the seething mass of living people with the attendant noise and smells of everyday life is more like the centre of a vast, bustling market place. There is no running water – just a few wells outside the building, and no toilets – just rows of pit latrines, built with help from Oxfam. No school for the children and not much play.*

*Life here is earnest and hopeful. There is no apathy in these people. They are all going about their business of making a fresh start for themselves and their children.*

*When a new family arrives in the camp, they usually have no possessions. A typical family will have lost the father, who may be a serving soldier, missing, killed, or taken prisoner. The mother and perhaps grandmother and grandfather, with from one to eight children, arrive – sometimes on foot or sometimes by ox-cart, army truck or canoe. They have just what they can carry: a very few clothes, a cooking pot, a water jar, a sleeping mat. They are all hungry, the babies crying.*

*First they must register with the camp chief, involving more anxiety and waiting – they cannot read or write – then they are allocated floor space – often the worst in the camp – wet, draughty and dirty, but at least a temporary refuge to rest in. They have never been in a city before – no cars or tuk-tuks in their village, nor foreigners. They've never seen so many people all at once – they are terrified. There is a weekly handout of food rations from the World Food Programme; they must cook their own once they get it. Their neighbours in the camp are generally kind to them and help them; they too were in the same situation a few days before so they know what it is like and they even may give a little of their precious rice ration to last the newcomers until the next handout. They show the mother their new 'relief bag' – with cooking pots, sleeping mats and water pot – provided by one or other foreign organisation or mission. They tell the family there is a soup kitchen where each child under sixteen years can get a free meal every morning and the health clinic where she can get free treatment for a sick child – even dried milk for a hungry baby. Mother sleeps on her floor space, now comforted that her children may have enough to survive.*

*Rice is given out to each camp family every week for the first three months in camp – after this time they are expected to have found some way to support themselves. A man may have found a paid job, working as a labourer or driving a rickshaw or even a tuk-tuk. Women may sell things on the street or in the main market. Within the camp small businesses have sprung up. One man has opened a shop and even employs three men. He makes wooden beds for families, if they can find wood. Several women have acquired hand sewing machines – often given by foreign organisations – and run their own dress-making business if material can be found. There are two small markets in camp, selling cooked food. Above all, there is a livestock business. These people are mostly farmers with livestock living around them – buffalo, cows, donkeys, oxen, pigs, goats, geese, ducks, chickens. (The latter are big business, especially ducks, which are a delicacy here. Eggs are hatched in cardboard boxes in the family space. Ducklings are guarded by the bigger boys and herded into the improvised farmyard at the back of the hotel – a very dirty place.)*

*Thus each little family settles into the miserable new life and gradually, hopefully, gets onto its feet again. A little money gets put by and, after a few months, thoughts turn to the possibility of going home or even resettlement somewhere in the city – a camp house or a tenement. Schools are all closed still.*

We found a small, but well-built, villa next door to the biggest 'camp' in The Casino Cambodiana. (This is now a luxury hotel on the banks of the Mekong River.) To this day I do not know who I approached to use the building, but they seemed like city officials. I think they were so pleased for us to help them with this huge problem that it was simplest for them to agree to our taking over not just one, but two adjacent villas. Thus began the Cambodiana health clinic and its daughter child-health clinic. What I didn't realise then was that being on the bank of the Mekong was not the safest location for us or our patients. We were very exposed to enemy fire across the river and we had several rocket hits over the years.

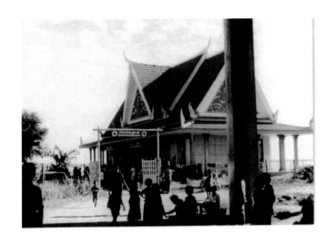

*World Vision Medical Clinic, 1973*

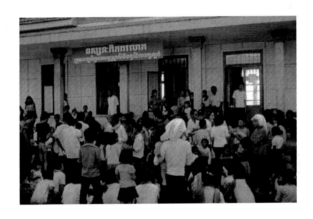

*Cambodiana Clinic – Waiting to get in*

But we set up our clinic with a large waiting area and two consulting rooms, one small laboratory, one injection room and a dispensary. This meant taking on more staff to run it. There was no shortage of applicants. There was little employment for young people and even qualified staff were not being paid. We quickly employed two young doctors (Dr Duong Sok Phan and Dr Kim Nguon), recently graduated and very keen. Also we found several nurses, a pharmacist and lab technician. We were a team of fifty already. This was not entirely to plan, but so much was needed that our World Vision employers soon agreed and appealed for funding from the public at home. Unfortunately, Dr Jim left us at that time. I know that he was not happy at the route we were following. He was tired and a good deal older than the rest of us. I valued the start he gave us and we missed his experience and wisdom, especially in relations with the local churches and government.

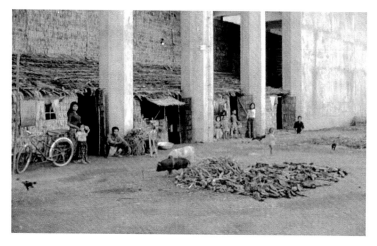

*Refugee homes under the hotel building*

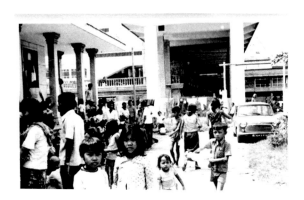

*Under the Cambodiana Hotel – and my Mini*

My next challenge was to find medicines and nutritious baby food. I went to all possible sources in Phnom Penh, which had a strong, expensive, but depleted, pharmaceutical industry. I had to fly off to Bangkok to get enough suitable medicines at a reasonable price. Most of the milk and high-calorie food substitutes came from the aid agencies – World Food Programme and USAID. We set up a small store and pharmacy at the back of our house and from there the young doctors supervised the sterilisation of our injection packs and the medicine boxes, which we took out daily to the clinics. It was a huge enterprise and required dedicated work from everyone. They enjoyed being useful and absorbed my daily medical and child health teaching with enthusiasm. I was helped throughout by the tireless commitment of Margaret, Joan and Mary Lou, who all brought ideas and energy to getting things set up and implemented.

We did not stop with just the one clinic. And although we were treating a thousand children and adults every day, we knew there were many more needing our care. So we went off to assess where and what to start.

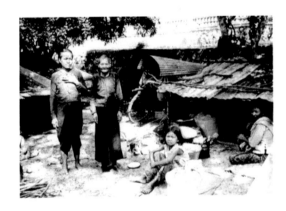

*A make-shift refugee house*

## IDP (Internally Displaced People) Camps

As fleeing people came into the city, the authorities were trying to put them into camps around the edge of the city. Cynically, we used to say that this made a barrier to the main population and that the enemy would 'get them' first. They certainly did later bear the brunt of rocket attacks.

World Vision was already involved in constructing emergency housing in the camps so it was relatively easy and obvious for us to send in a medical team. Thus started our mobile clinics, which did a huge amount of work every day. The first camp clinic we opened was at Pochentong, near the main airport, followed closely by Km 12 and Obaykam Camp clinics.

# Other Non-Government Organisations (NGOs)

The NGOs – for example International Red Cross, Save the Children Fund, SE Asian Outreach, CARE, Evangelical Alliance, and others – were very important at that time. National health services had been virtually destroyed. There were still some city hospitals supposed to be functioning. In reality, they had no medicines and little equipment. Under the French system, every province had one referral hospital, with health centres and posts at village level and manned by paramedics and nurses. These had mostly disappeared through lack of pay, maintenance or staff. What was left at village level were traditional healers and midwives or sometimes private doctors. The prevalent infectious diseases – malaria, tuberculosis and leprosy – increased dangerously, and both maternal and child mortality was extremely high.

# Embassies

Interestingly, we were given not inconsiderable help from ladies of the embassies. They supported our work through donations of infant food, clothing and sometimes volunteers. The US Embassy in particular was very supportive and I often talked at their ladies' meetings.

# Our progress

Meanwhile our clinics grew and grew, both at the Cambodiana Clinic and our camp mobiles. We had difficulties over transport. We simply did not have enough. We were allocated an old Land Rover and a minibus. That meant drivers and more money. We were proving expensive to World Vision Australia and had to supplement our fundraising from our homes. Margaret brought in lots from her family's efforts. I sought my mother and father's help from home. They both appealed to their old friends and parishioners. My old parish church at Highweek had a huge fund-raising event which they called 'Pennies for Pene' – laying a mile of pennies around the church and village. I was able to assure them that their pennies were very well spent.

I used funds from home to buy food and medicines from Thailand. The support from home was highly valued. Then I was able to get WV to buy me my own car. It made a huge difference to my mobility and clinic supervision. I bought a bright orange Mini from the British Embassy. It had been imported for a staff member who did not then want it. I snapped it up and was then highly visible and well known by the soldiers throughout the city as I zipped around from camp to clinic and hospitals and home. It was especially valuable when the curfews started. As soon as the dry season started in December, the enemy came close to the city and infiltrated the borders. A night curfew was imposed by the national army/police – from 7.00 pm to 7.00 am. If we ventured outside, we were stopped and cautioned: it was not allowed. I regularly disobeyed the curfew because of patient care, but my orange Mini usually meant a quick wave-through from the soldiers and police, who often removed the barriers for me. I kept my Mini until I left Phnom Penh in April 1975 and, sadly, I never found it again – though I had a good look after my return years later.

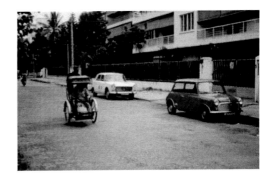

*My orange Mini on a street outside my flat in Phnom Penh*

## Triage at the Cambodiana Clinic

Some days when we started work at the clinic, we could not get in for pressure of people. We were almost mobbed by mothers trying to push in to be registered for examination by our doctors.

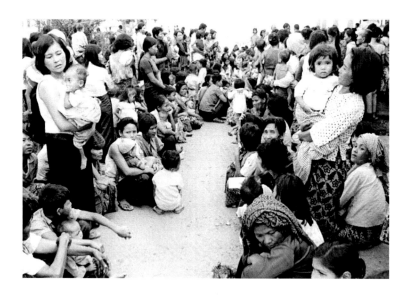

*Morning Queue*

It was a big worry to know how to choose the worst cases and to stop relatively well people from taking up our time and energy. We gave it much thought and discussion together. The decision was to try a triage system. This meant we needed frontline staff to choose those from the crowd to be brought to see the doctors. Our doctors needed training too. They were not used to treating children in this state and they knew little about malnutrition. So I remained the last in the line when they could not cope. This kept me busy every day. We trained our most experienced male nurses to front the triage. What a task they had! Faced with long lines of distraught mothers with very ill children, the nurses had to pick out the ones they considered most in need of help and put a mark on them to allow them to be registered in the clinic. The people soon got to understand the system we operated and how to copy the mark. When we were faced with a relatively well, fat baby, we knew that the system was not working. We changed the marks daily and even had a special ink stamp made, but it was still copied. It was the best we could do and even then some slipped through. I can still see and hear in my dreams the thousands of women and children waiting at the gate for us to arrive every morning, and see their faces when we packed up every evening and left them unseen for another day.

106

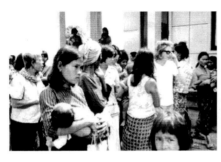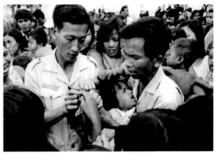

*Triage at the clinic*                          *Fighting for the triage mark*

The next problem I had not anticipated was how to keep our staff – and ourselves – healthy. Now recognised as an issue for disaster aid workers, no one had thought of it in our day. I quickly knew that I was losing weight fast, but that was good for me and did not worry me at all. It was impossible to eat or drink in the clinic; every child and most women were starving and any snacks we had went to them. Cambodians take their lunch break seriously and eat their main meal at midday. So we did take a break for two hours. We ourselves had lunch cooked for us at our home. Our doctors came to me one day and said how worried they were that the staff, including themselves, were not getting good food at lunchtime, because they had no transport to go home. They had little energy to work through the afternoon. We had a re-think and finally agreed to provide a hot meal for any staff who really needed it. Disappointingly, this lunch became a source of complaint as staff thought we gave them a second-class meal — not well cooked. We could not seem to do the right thing and a compromise was reached when we sent them out to buy food in the market. My Thivan watched me closely and spoke firmly to me when she thought I needed food and watched to make sure I did not give it away. We bought crates of bottled drinks to re-hydrate us all.

Our patients had many infections which were all too easy to pick up. For us expatriates, diarrhoea and dysentery were our big problem and we went down one after another. I had a nasty bout of typhoid fever and was off work for a couple of weeks. When I was ill, I was very worried when my staff, including the doctors, would not leave me alone in peace. Actually, I did not much like it and used to ask them to leave me. I know better now.

107

Thivan soon explained to me that they were all worried lest I died alone. They stayed close so that they could call my spirit back if it went away. So I went along with them each time I was ill, though I do not think I was ever near to death at all.

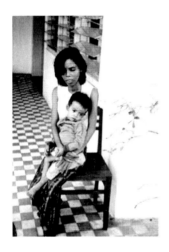

*Mother and a very ill child*
*waiting for their turn*

## Tuol Kork Nutrition Centre (TKNC)

I had been treating children in developing countries for more than ten years but I had never seen anything like this. It was very soon evident that there was a food crisis (WHO did not agree) and that the children were starving. I used to describe the situation as acute or chronic under-nutrition. The young under-five year group were almost without exception suffering from protein deficiency as well as vitamin deficiencies – especially vitamin A. On top of this already precarious state, they were now plunged into an acute phase, which showed itself as marasmus and kwashiorkor. The only treatment for this was food — mainly protein and vitamins. The small babies were in a bad way, as most mothers had little or no breast milk as they too were starving. If they did manage to buy or find a baby's feeding bottle, they had nothing to put in it. Baby milk powder was off the market, but they had no money anyway. I have a haunting memory of a young mother holding out for me her very young baby and clutching a murky-looking solution in a dirty feeding bottle. I asked her, through Thivan, what was in the mixture. She told me, 'Water mixed with sand, to fill her up, but now she has stomach pains.' How desperate do you have to be to scrape dirt off the ground and feed it to your baby?

The question for us was 'what to do'? It was useless to hand out medicines: they needed food. So we set up feeding centres in the camps and clinics. We had two levels. The nurses screened out the children needing feeding urgently. They gave advice, and milk powder in plastic bags. We received a lot of criticism for this from other NGOs like Save the Children Fund. We knew very well the arguments against doing this (bottle-feeding killing babies through infection from dirty water). But we decided to try – we would save some. We taught the mothers to cup- and spoon-feed the babies and children, to avoid the dirty water and bottle problem. What we brought upon ourselves then was the problem of sheer numbers. Word got round fast that we gave out free milk. Mothers came flocking to us. How to choose and how to refuse some? The problem was most critical at the nutrition centre we set up at the Cambodiana camp, next to our health clinic. Here we had decided to admit the worst children for the day, along with mothers or elder sisters (who were often deputed as the baby/toddler carer and who were highly receptive to our teaching). The advantage for me was that this centre was nearby so I could do a daily round to look at the children. The frustration was that we did not have the children for evenings and nights, and so never knew if they would turn up again next day.

## Staff

I need to go back a little: my expatriate team was getting tired through the unceasing pressure of work. We asked Australia for more staff, especially nurses with nutrition experience. Margaret and I were developing an idea to do more for undernourished children. We realised they needed round-the-clock care if they were to survive. In consultation with our director and funders, we started looking around for a large house where we could open a centre. We joyfully accepted an Australian nurse with excellent paediatric nursing experience to help us. Sandra Menz duly arrived in our second year. Sandra had had a serious illness but still had a calling to give service at the front line with us. Together we assessed the situation and opened a nutrition centre for undernourished children in a large villa in Tuol Kork – a city suburb on the airport road. It opened its doors in October 1974.

*Below: A selection of pictures taken at Tuol Kork Nutrition Centre*

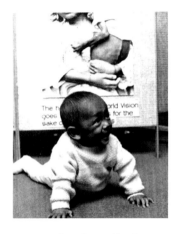

*Orphan Carl*

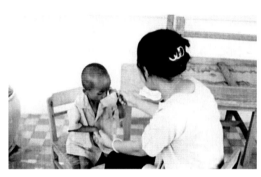

*An abandoned child*

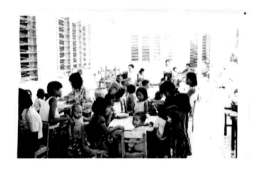

*Dinner time*

*Pene with a child in the Tuol Kork Nutrition Centre*

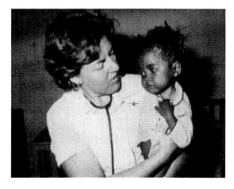

110

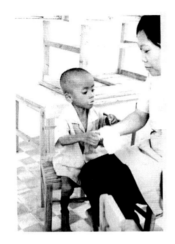

*Starving child – a chance to eat*

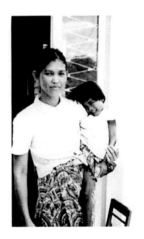

*Going home well*

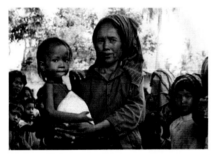

*Mother and child with milk bag as distributed at camps*

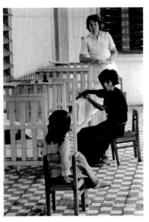

*Nutrition Ward*

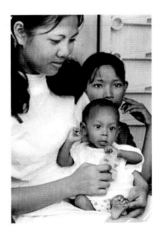

*Orphans getting better*

111

Our lives now changed significantly. All our nurses were involved with teaching and/or caring at the TKNC.

As for myself, I had to do a daily ward round – sometimes twice or more when children were very ill. We took on more Cambodian staff to cover the added workload, and Dr Kim Nguon was almost full-time as medical cover. He was a caring doctor, loved by us all. He learned from Sandra and me the essentials of the care of such children.

We had good back-up from Dr Beat Richner and even referred children to his hospital if we thought he could do more than us. We concentrated our efforts on nutrition care and watched with delight when the kwashiorkor children ate their way to good health again. The biggest problem we faced was other infections. For instance, measles went through the camps and our centre – with devastating mortality. Many young children had tuberculosis, and typhoid made a deadly appearance. The night curfew meant that none of us expats could provide medical cover at night. Many tragic mornings we arrived at TKNC to be greeted by several little bundles wrapped in cotton cloths –sometimes three or four patients had given up the struggle in the night. Then we had to discover about going to the temples for traditional cremation and the monk's prayers for the deceased. No concessions were made for those without money – or even for babies – and so, of course, we paid the bill.

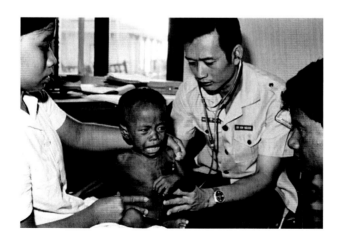

*Dr Nguon*

# Orphans

From the beginning we faced the issue of abandoned babies. Men were now serving in one army or another – as conscripts or volunteers. Women were left at home in the villages with no means of support. In their village economy, both men and women had their allotted tasks. Women planted the rice fields but men usually harvested it, and certainly transported the grain from the fields to the grain stores for husking. Without the men, the women were left without new rice and faced starvation for themselves and their children. New babies were just an extra burden to be breast-fed as long as possible, thus weakening the mother. But after weaning, the mother faced finding food for the extra mouth and with no future for the child anyway, if a chance came up to hand over the baby, even to a foreigner, it would be taken readily. The women were getting to know and trust us all and to them we were rich beyond imagining. They saw us caring for babies and feeding children all day, every day – so why not their kids? – and they started to walk away when we were treating or feeding a sick baby. While we had the TK nutrition centre, the babies could be absorbed among the patients there, fed and loved by our nurses and all staff. It was different with bigger children.

There were thousands of children on the streets of Phnom Penh at that time. Most had no homes, and little to eat except what they managed to beg or steal. A few, initially just two or three, ended up living in our house. None of us was prepared to turn a young child from our clinic onto the streets. I soon gathered a little flock and we made a dormitory at the back of our house and allowed them to sleep there and share our food. We were pressurised to hand them over to local orphanages – but life there was miserable and we could not do it. One or two mothers turned up to claim a child, but this was rare. One little boy sticks in my mind even now. I found him wandering around outside the clinic. He was about ten years old and he would not speak. He had a blank, shuttered face but did not cry. Our female staff gradually got a story from him and it was awful. His mother and family had been killed one night in a rocket attack. He survived and walked away into the city, totally on his own. He was scared out of his mind. We gave him love, food and shelter. He started to eat and even play again, but never lost that look of fear. He lost his childhood like so many others there at that time.

By mid-1974, we had fourteen children living at our house – known now as Penny's children, but they were everybody's as they came in from every clinic, not just mine. It was lovely to have them around and I think they helped us to keep things in perspective and de-stress us. Ever since that time, I have resolved to always keep a child in my life. I believe it is a good resolve for all of us who are single and getting older. A child not only keeps you young, but also keeps you interested in the young world and in matters beyond yourself. Of course, a hungry or unloved child is even easier for one to love.

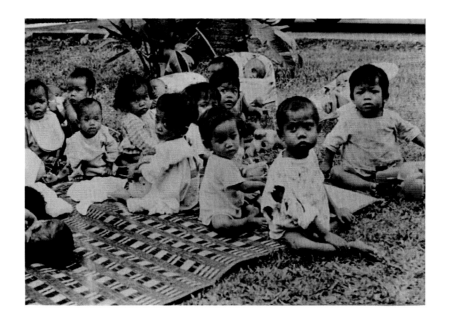

*Our Orphans*

# Chapter 5: Deteriorating situation in Cambodia

## Security

Meanwhile, in the autumn of 1973, the Khmer Rouge was advancing on Phnom Penh. The rains had been huge and there was flooding across the plain around the city. The dry season offensive came in literally with a bang. We had to start taking security very seriously – for ourselves and our patients. We were given many directions and advice from our embassies and international agencies. Our patients in the clinic told us that the enemy was infiltrating the city and our staff were convinced that we were treating enemy soldiers in our clinic. From the beginning, we had banned guns and arms in the clinic building, but this did not deter uniformed soldiers in groups. They ruled the roost and could make demands.

One day in the clinic I was made aware of a disturbance in the waiting area. I went out to investigate. My staff, including Dr Sokphan, were highly agitated and pulling agony faces at me – I did not know why. I saw a young man in khaki, clutching his belt and gesturing for medicines and milk to be handed over. When I appeared, someone must have said that I was in charge, as he at once turned to me and demanded treatment. I was angry. I saw no reason to give him anything so I refused and told him to leave – which he did very quickly. When he left, my staff surrounded me saying, 'No, he was not ill.' So my reputation of being immune to danger started. I went through a good many 'nears' over the next two years – incidents that I did not write home about. Sometimes I was very scared but I knew I was being looked after for a purpose and had a big task ahead of me.

## Incidents and near misses in Cambodia – the first year

Incoming rockets were the main danger that first dry season. The enemy had pushed up the far bank of the Mekong River until they were almost opposite us. Then they started firing their long-range rockets. These came whooshing over our heads, high and low – but always fell somewhere within the city, doing damage where they landed. They always came in threes, following each other at intervals of about five seconds. My first encounter with a rocket was when I was in my car being driven by a faithful Khmer driver (Samol) when we stopped suddenly to see a rocket whoosh across our path ahead, almost touching the bonnet. Instead of stopping, Samol put his foot down hard on the accelerator shouting, 'There will be two more – it's safer to get away.' He was right and we were unharmed, though shocked and thankful for being spared. I owed my life to Samol, who did not survive Pol Pot.

## Rockets at our clinic

Not many days later, I was standing outside the Cambodiana Clinic, conducting the daily triage, when a rocket almost 'parted my hair'. I instinctively went flat on my face but was immediately pulled to my feet by a team member, Beng On (from Singapore), who shouted, 'Get in there!' and pointed to a nearby crater left by the rocket. Soon I found myself lying in the hole alongside Beng On and asking, 'Why here?' He said, 'Rockets always come in threes, but one never falls exactly where the first landed.' It seemed true enough, as two more rockets screamed in above our heads and exploded a few yards further away, but too near to the baby feeding clinic for my liking. Soon screaming women came running from the camp to find their babies – none harmed, praise God. But we learned to be more careful.

In the same month, schools in Phnom Penh took direct hits, one being destroyed, along with many young children, by six rockets. This had a huge impact on our expatriate community as several families we knew suffered losses.

In 1974, as the rains came down, the Khmer Rouge army started to withdraw from frontline activity and we all breathed freely again and increased our services outside the city. Planes and helicopters started to fly out around the country without the constant fear of being shot down. American aid agencies were leading the relief at this time and several times they came to me to ask for a medical team to go out and visit one particular town or camp where they had found great suffering.

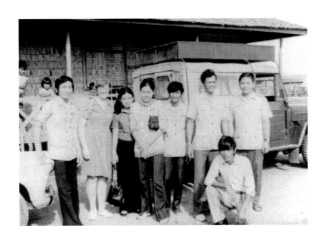

*Emergency mobile medical team 1974 (Thivan with her handbag)*

I remember travelling with two medical teams out to Pursat and Konpong Cham to treat ill people in health centres or non-functional hospitals. It was a welcome change to get away from our clinic routine in the city and to begin to see the Cambodian countryside, even though it showed evidence of the war and destruction, but we always knew the enemy was still there, although in hiding. We knew because the villagers told us horror stories most days at the clinics. One memorable day at the Km 6 Dyke Camp, there was a large group of very distressed women with children. We had not seen them before. We heard they had arrived only that morning. After a bit, the Cambodian staff got the terrible story. In the late evening the Khmer Rouge had attacked their village, less than 20 km up the river from us. The village men tried to resist attack and to fight, whereupon the soldiers killed all the men and boys, cut off their heads and threw the heads into the river in front of the women. They then drove the women out of the village, threatening death to the children and women too if they resisted. The women were still convinced the enemy were following and were not far away from us. Sure enough, we could hear gunfire not far away and getting nearer. We continued the clinic, but after a short time the Khmer staff begged us to close down and leave. We did not want to, but better safe than dead, so we packed up and prepared to go home in our vulnerable jeeps. I remember that we could not find Margaret. She had no intention of running away and would not leave the needy women just because of gunfire. At the very last minute, the Khmer staff went and grabbed her, forcing her into a vehicle. She was not happy but I was most relieved.

## War stepping up

Because reports of enemy progress in the country increased, embassies started to wind down and even to close. Most, including the US and UK, sent all women and children out, leaving the staff alone to battle through. There were quite a lot of staff still in the country and we were permitted to stay, but had to respect embassy instructions on where we could work and travel. Being a mostly female expat team, we found ourselves a focus for social invitations and for concern. I was sent for regularly to brief the British ambassador on the health and social situation. It was rather pleasant to escape from the pressures of clinics to the calm of the Embassy. I remember an incredible Christmas dinner in 1974 on the roof of the British Residence, when, during the sweet course after a traditional Christmas feast (including all the trimmings and good French wine), the inevitable happened: rockets started coming in and round us, too close for comfort. We all looked to HE (His Excellency) for instructions, but he, in a most English way, stood up, saying, 'Ladies and Gentlemen, shall we take our coffee downstairs?' We all thankfully descended to relative safety, and no damage was sustained.

I also vividly remember the German counsellor and his wine-tasting. He was a remarkable man – a baron in Germany. He loved Cambodia dearly and had built a store of fine German wines, shipping them from home to sail up the Mekong River on barges to Phnom Penh port. By this time, the Mekong was mostly under the control of the Khmer Rouge soldiers, and cargo ships never made the port, except for those carrying the German wine, right up to the last year. So my colleagues and I got invited to surreal parties to taste the latest arrivals. It was quite an experience to sit in the garden being served with bread, cheese and wines. It was all done in the correct professional way and we were seriously taught (in this time of war) how to discern fine wine, as if it were the most crucial thing to know just then. It brought a real sparkle to our lives and I will always be grateful to the baron, who I hear is now an ambassador somewhere.

The British Red Cross surgical team lived in a house next door to ours. They were good neighbours who always helped us. At this time, nights were becoming very noisy and more dangerous as the intensity of firing became more frequent, more accurate and louder. Many nights we all congregated downstairs in our house, sleeping all together on the marble floor, in the shelter of a strong wall. It was not restful. Very early one morning our guard came running, shouting that the house next door had been hit in the night. We knew there had been many hits close by, but this was disaster and we went to find our friends. A rocket had entered through the bedroom window of one of the British nurses. She had moved out of her bed and gone downstairs, like us. The bed suffered a direct hit and there was not much left for her in that room. None of the team were hurt and they just got on with their jobs – an inspiring example to us. Later, a British doctor on their team came and told us that he had been walking down the street when he started hearing the customary screech of rockets; one hit a tree on the pavement where he was. The tree was split in pieces and came down beside him and he walked on very shaken, but unhurt.

I could continue with many more stories but must move on with our team's story. I have now reached the end of our first dry-season offensive, after which we got ourselves much better organised and meeting a bigger need in the growing camps. The fighting in the countryside displaced many more thousands of people. And the camps of displaced people in and around the city grew. Malnutrition and disease abounded among the children, and numbers in the TK nutrition centre went up and up. At that time we were sent a team of nurses and a doctor from New Zealand. They were very young and idealistic. They found it hard to fit into the disaster medicine we were undertaking and the young doctor thought we were not treating the patients as we should, or according to his medical training. He worked hard for a bit, but finally could not cope and went home – to my sorrow.

We were being warned that there would be a major push in the next (1974) dry season. We even took part in emergency evacuation practices, not really believing we would have to experience a real one.

# Evacuation

At the beginning of the dry season in late 1974, the British Embassy decided to send all children and women (including workers) home. This would include Australians, New Zealanders and Indians, because Britain was looking after their interests. The Ambassador sent for me one day and said he had a problem and please would I help him. His female staff and some British Aid agency staff (Save the Children Fund, OXFAM, etc.) were refusing to leave. He anticipated, rightly, that my staff might do likewise. He wanted me to announce I was going out and others should follow my lead. I saw his point but was most unhappy. In fact, I said I would consider and get back to him. I went straight to my colleagues in the US Embassy. We were looking after a lot of their people by then. I told them my problem and asked them whether, if I returned after evacuation, they would put me under their umbrella for security purposes. I was not quite brave enough to snap my fingers at all of them and have no one to run to. We were all quite frightened of flying now. Rockets were regularly hitting the airport and clearly the enemy were not far away. Would any planes get in or out without being shot down? I agreed to the Ambassador that if he could organise an evacuation, I would go along and look after the evacuees. I don't know how many I influenced – not many, I think. From my own team, two Australians gave up and went out, but not all – and certainly not Margaret. We had word from the British Embassy that next morning a British army plane would come in to take us out. We could join the Embassy vehicles to travel out to Pochentong Airport. Now, whenever I land or take off from the same airport, I remember with thanks what happened that day, which was an unforgettable experience.

# Pochentong

It was a normal hot, sunny day in the summer season. Barbed wire and soldiers surrounded Pochentong Airport. There were army planes and helicopters under camouflage nets at the far end of the runway. Our little group, with the British Ambassador, and a posse of young women and small children, were huddled in the old VIP lounge awaiting instructions and were all rather scared. We could hear gunfire not far away. After a while, some official ran in and said to the ambassador, 'Your planes are coming in now.' We ran to windows to try to see, but it wasn't until we were escorted out onto the tarmac that we saw two Hercules aeroplanes with Union Jacks parked at the far side of the airport runway. We were all escorted in old buses, with our luggage, across to the planes. Each Hercules had the back door open and ramps in place. The Ambassador told me, 'Pene, you go first and then they will follow,' so I did.

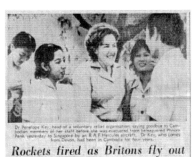
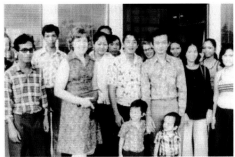

*Rockets fired as Britons fly out*

*Airport good-byes*

What an incongruous bunch we were, along with prams, babies and endless bundles and bags pouring into the belly of the plane. There weren't any seats, as we understand them. There was webbing as used for troop-carrying. No one was used to this but we were wanting to get away before the enemy got a fix on us. Then rockets starting coming in. I vividly remember sheltering under a wing alongside the Ambassador. Flat on the ground, he had a hard hat on, but I did not. Eventually we got everyone seated and gave the OK to the crew to go. But there was more to come. I learned that the crew were three very young Irish army recruits. They had never been under fire and were terrified. They had been diverted from a routine leave flight to Singapore to come in and pick us up. They knew nothing of the war here and didn't know what to do. Someone summoned me to the cockpit. I tried to fill them in briefly with what was going on, the main items being that the rockets were fired randomly from the west of the airport, that they always came in salvos of three and then a gap of about five minutes before the next salvo. We needed to wait for one lot and then take off quickly to the south. So I stood behind the pilot officer counting rockets; 'One, two, three – they did not hit us. Go, go, go!' We've taken off, but what was the bang on the plane? Oh, it was just a tyre bursting – no matter. The young men sweated, white and shaking, and all of us felt pretty relieved.

The plane set course for Singapore and we all relaxed as we went up and out of range of the guns and rockets. We had contacted Singapore and been told we would be met and looked after there by staff from the Embassy. When we got near Singapore, the pilot got worried and said to his crew, 'How many tyres do you think we burst taking off?' No one knew and he could only radio ahead and warn Singapore we might have a difficult landing.

We did indeed have a bad landing. As we touched down, all the tyres seemed to explode. They said afterwards that they must all have been hit by gunfire as we left. However, all was well and we were soon bussed in to the calm and safety of Singapore International Airport – a different world indeed! Families were given food, drinks and allocated rooms in a hotel nearby. We all had to sign papers agreeing that we would pay our onward airfare to our home countries if asked. At the time, there were a lot of complaints about this – but everyone signed anyway. Respective embassies took over care of their citizens. I never did see a British representative but was under the care of Australians. From my hotel room that night I rang home, saying, 'I'm out, but going back.' My mother was not impressed. I had no idea then how I would go back. All I could think of were the children I should be treating back home in Phnom Penh.

Next morning I went to the airport and bought a ticket to Bangkok as the main route to Phnom Penh. It did not take long. I had a lot of contacts in Bangkok then and I seem to remember that I went off at once to the Christian Guest House in central Bangkok. It felt like home and they were all very kind to me in my rather distraught state. I called Phnom Penh and asked Carl how I could get back, as there were no commercial flights at that time. He said, 'Try the US Embassy,' which I did next morning. I was surprised that they seemed unsurprised to hear from me (perhaps they had heard from Carl) and they offered me a seat on a US army supply Hercules that afternoon. That was wonderful and, before I could even go shopping, I was out to the airport again and onto another plane. It was an easy flight and I loved arriving again at the airport and being greeted by rather scared team members, who I suspect really would rather I had stayed away from the danger.

## Our house

Back at 10 Keo Chea, all was rather 'jittery'; the house next door had been hit and there was no telling where the rockets would land next, but we did seem to be protected to do our job each day. There were many camps that were now out of bounds for security reasons and we had to re-programme our teams. We also had to carry emergency kits in case of rocket accidents. I recall one: an airport camp we visited had received a rocket attack in the night and there were injuries – no one knew how bad.

## The media

The international media were in attendance and causing problems. I went myself, with our team, to give medical help. There was chaos and no other medical help except us. An injured man was brought to our emergency shelter in an old hut. He had received a hit from a large piece of shrapnel that was lodged under his arm and he was haemorrhaging badly. My nurses and I did what we could but clearly he needed surgery to stop the bleeding. I had to try to do something on the spot otherwise he would have died. I remember it was very dark and I could only see anything when a press man took a photo with a flash. So I asked the camera men to help to set up a flashlight focus on the upper arm so that I could find the bleeding spot. It was very difficult, but I got there in the end and clamped the pulsing artery with small forceps. Then we bundled him up and took him to the Red Cross in the hospital. I doubt he survived.

My relations with the press at that time were good – I think because I always told a story and was willing to talk to them – on my terms. At this late stage, there were always masses of cameras and press men waiting at the Cambodiana Clinic in the early mornings to get photos of the masses of mothers and sick children waiting for us. I was rather firm with the reporters. In fact, I could have upset them when I bargained with them, even eminent names such as The Times and The Daily Telegraph – and the American press. I said I would give one interview per day and not more; how could I, with so many patients waiting? I said they could share and I could talk to several together, but would not be available more than once. They accepted this and I found myself being interviewed by these famous news reporters on all human aspects of the present situation. Then I asked for their help and they gave it. I said I was not happy for them just to stand around taking pictures when there was so much to be done. Please would they help our staff to sort people out, give medicines out, hold children, etc? They were marvellous and set to willingly. I remember a reporter helping me with a very ill child, acting as a drip-stand, holding up the bottle of saline while I inserted the needle. I think they were happy to be of use. They certainly got good pictures.

Then I had to say goodbye to 'our' children. There was no guarantee that we could stay and it was no longer safe for the fourteen children in our house. Margaret and I searched around looking for a safe place for them. Eventually we arranged to transfer them to an orphanage in the city, where there was support being given to the children by an American agency. The children seemed well cared for. So they sadly left us and I never knew what happened to them – but fear the worst, given what happened to all vulnerable people.

\*\*\*

In late 1974, when the dry season offensive was in full swing and we were all extremely busy feeding hundreds of starving children and treating all manner of tropical diseases – malaria, typhoid, dysentery, measles and gunshot wounds – one day I wrote the following piece for the World Vision magazine:

## 'Why must there be a choice?' by Dr Penelope Key,

### Director, World Vision Medical Team

Today I waved goodbye to a little Cambodian girl (Becca) leaving her native country for her new home and family in America.

124

Beside me, my Cambodian doctor colleague said, 'She is a lucky, lucky little girl. Why did she get chosen?'

Today, in my clinic at the Cambodian refugee centre, there were more than 500 mothers with their sick children, waiting for their turn. Some will come again tomorrow, and some the next day. I chose 200-300 children from among them. The rest are not chosen. There is agony for me in this choosing. When I put up my hand at the end of a five-hour morning's stretch – when I call to my doctors, nurses and clerks, 'That child is the last one for the morning,' what am I doing or saying to the child after the last one? The anguish of the mother whose child is refused haunts me and my staff. Her face stays with us as we eat our lunch, knowing that she is waiting and watching her child.

Sometimes a waiting child dies while I am away resting. How then can I rest – or eat or sleep? How can I not choose to see that child? Why did I choose to stop at the child before that one? If I had chosen to see one more child, that child might be alive today.

This morning there were 34 children needing admission to the hospital. There were only seven empty cots. I had to choose. Twenty-seven critically ill children went to their homes in the arms of their despairing mothers.

Bob, in your letter from Bangladesh (December 1974 issue, pp. 4-7), you say you can help one mother, one father, one child, one at a time. I can only help one at a time, too. How do I choose which one? All these children are God's little ones. He loves and cares about every one of them. I believe He wants every one of them to be cared for. He does not want me to choose one from another. He loves them all. I have a prayer I use: Lord, don't let me have to go on choosing which child. Lord, send me more doctors. Lord, send me more cots, more hospitals, more medicines, milk and food. Lord, give all these children enough food so they won't get sick. Lord, please stop this senseless war.

Becca was chosen from a line of sick children in my clinic. Did I choose her? Did God choose her? Or is she just an exceedingly

125

fortunate little girl?  When can all my children be chosen for a new, happy life?  – Will it really be happy for them?'

\*\*\*

I met Becca again in the USA when she was 15 years old.  She had become a little American, adopted into a family of four boys.  She was greatly loved but had not settled well into school life.  She found it all very difficult socially.  She knew she was different but did not understand her origins.  She never wanted to go back – unless she has changed her mind since.  I know she married very young – an Afro-American.  I hope her life is settled and happy.  I hope I made a difference for her.

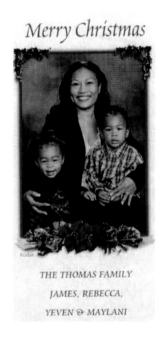

### Merry Christmas

THE THOMAS FAMILY
JAMES, REBECCA,
YEVEN & MAYLANI

*Rebecca's family, Christmas 18 years later.*
*Rebecca is the orphan girl Becca I rescued – she was nearly starving.*

\*\*\*

## Airport evacuation

We listened avidly to news of the Vietnam war on the BBC World Service or other radio, such as American and French stations. It always got much more coverage internationally than Cambodia, and we knew when things were really bad there because we did not get enough planes in to feed the city people. By this stage of our war, there was famine in Phnom Penh. There just was nothing in the markets even if one had money. All birds had long since been eaten; cats and dogs were now hunted and eaten. The Americans led the operation to feed everyone. I remember a meeting called by the International Red Cross to work out the logistics of providing relief feeding to the people.

In retrospect, I wonder why the official government agencies were not involved, but at that time they were all in disarray. Many Cambodian leaders had left the country in fear; others were keeping a low profile and trying to escape with their families. We were proud when Carl Harris on our behalf offered World Vision services to set up a feeding programme for almost half the city. It meant re-deploying our medical teams to the feeding programme, but it was good in that our staff knew the people and were known. Our staff all worked so hard and willingly, when they too were frightened because of the daily bombardment. We distributed rice and flour in bags. This was all flown in from Saigon (now Ho Chi Minh City) in US army planes. We watched them flying in over the city every day – we almost 'counted them in and counted them out'. It would have been too easy for them to get hit by gunfire or rockets but it seemed they were lucky – as were we. We reckoned that around 30 planes came in every day. Then the number started to fall. The watchers reported only 25 planes one day and then only 20. Then the rice began to run out. We learned afterwards that the planes could not safely take off from Saigon Airport, let alone fly safely over Cambodia; and the city began to starve. We felt guilty about eating our protected rations.

*** 

Then one day in April 1975, we listened in disbelief to the evacuation of Americans from Vietnam. I think we knew then, in our hearts, that Cambodia would go the same way and that our days were numbered. We packed our cases and had them at the ready. In our house only Margaret and I remained. Carl was still in Phnom Penh heading up the World Vision relief operation, helped by many faithful Cambodian staff.

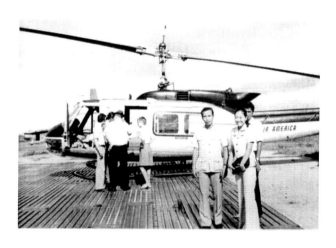

*A UN flight 1975 – Thivan with her handbag again*

The city was under constant bombardment now and each day it got worse; we were really frightened. Not many patients came to the clinics as they were scared to come out. I held one clinic at Pochentong health centre, near the airport. I sat at my consulting desk as usual, when rockets came in very near. I made everyone get down on the floor under a thick wall and made a dive there myself as another rocket screamed in and hit our centre. We all felt the blast but were not hit. When we could get up, one of my nurses said, 'Quick, come and see.' My desk had been blown apart and there was a large hole in it. If I had been sitting there instead of cowering by the wall, I would not have lived. This gave me confidence that I was not going to die; that there was work for me to do still. We received messages that the last passenger plane would likely take off next morning and we, the remaining expatriate foreign staff, would be on it. I had considerable confidence in my Cambodian staff now and knew I could rely on them to continue to provide medical care as long as possible. But Margaret and I both felt very guilty – how could we abandon them? What would happen to them? We talked through the options with them and they all insisted that we should depart. After all, they argued, the Khmer Rouge were fellow-Cambodians, not foreigners – so they would be safe!

The unforgettable day of 12th April 1975 dawned and Carl picked us up to go to the airport to catch our last plane. Simultaneously, we knew from all the commotion in town that the US Embassy was evacuating by helicopter.

There was massive gunfire overhead as the enemy tried to shoot down helicopters. We knew that soon their guns would be trained on our plane. Out at Pochentong Airport, there was chaos and lots of tears. We were each individually issued with a special boarding pass – non-transferable. There were lots of foreigners trying to get onto this last plane and tickets were very limited. I had two people after my boarding pass. One was a desperate young woman and I very nearly gave her my seat. I did not much want to leave anyway. But if I did not board the plane, I knew that Margaret would not – and probably Carl – how could I do this to them? So I meekly got on. I sat on the floor, there being no seats left. Eventually our plane took off, dodging the gunfire. I cowered on the floor, asking too often, 'Where are we? Have we left Cambodia yet?' The too-heavily-loaded plane rose very slowly and circled around maddeningly, to gain height. At long last it headed away en route to Bangkok, which is not far by direct route. After what seemed an age, I called out, 'Where are we now? Can you see Bangkok?' A voice answered me, 'No. I can still see Pochentong.' So we could still be hit. But after about 45 minutes we got there and landed safely at Bangkok International Airport, amidst loud cheering from us all. What a motley, scruffy crowd of passengers we must have looked to the Thai officials at the airport. When we came to the immigration desks, I remember cowering down, trying to pretend I had all my papers. I did not. The Thai officials insisted that we all needed visas to enter – not just our British passport. They argued that the Thai Embassy was still open in Phnom Penh (it was not) and we would have to go back there to get visas. How ridiculous! Meanwhile our baggage had been offloaded and was spotted the other side by our World Vision staff sent to meet us. Among them was Graham Irvine, Australia Director and my boss. Having identified us in our plight, he set about sorting out our problem and soon we were on our way into Thailand – on short-entry visas. My parents told me afterwards that they had no idea where I was or what was happening, except that things were very bad in Cambodia, until they saw footage of the evacuation. My red suitcase, which they had given me, appeared in a shot and that was how they knew that I (and my case) was out. I was able to speak to them later that day.

Then we had a debrief with Graham and the World Vision International Director, Stan Mooneyham. Both were very upset and I had the feeling that they would have preferred one of us to stay in Phnom Penh rather than 'run away'. We told them about all the babies and toddlers in our Tuol Kork centre; immediately they said, 'We must get them out.' I did not believe they meant it, but they did. Before I knew what was happening, I was booked onto a chartered plane next day to return to Phnom Penh and bring out staff families and as many orphaned children as we could carry from the centre. Margaret insisted on coming with me, but Carl had had enough. Graham and Stan both came, fully fitted out with tin hats and flak jackets.

\*\*\*

I was much more frightened this time. I felt that it was tempting fate to fly back into the inferno and especially to move a lot of children out. Quite recently there had been an awful air crash of a planeful of orphans which crashed taking off from Saigon. Before leaving Bangkok I had to speak on a radio link to Dr Sokphan to tell him we were coming and that he should prepare all the orphan babies and small children for us to carry out on our plane. He was amazed and not altogether happy. My instructions were, 'Send only orphans, and send only those fit to travel, not any seriously ill.' I left the details to him. 'Bring them to the airport ready to load onto the plane quickly for a speedy turnaround.'

So we landed again at Pochentong. It was still under heavy fire and we all donned tin hats and even flak jackets. We taxied to the terminal building and then saw all the white World Vision vehicles lined up on the tarmac. They were loaded with children and our staff. The plan was for each of us to go and carry a child into the plane. In the event, our staff carried the babies, all strapped into Moses baskets, and then the toddlers in their arms. Margaret and I, whom the children knew, helped bring them on board and settled them down. It was highly emotional for us. We had already said goodbye once and this was almost too much. Then there was another family loaded, the wife and children of Minh Voan (acting WV Director). He would not leave, himself, but he wanted his children out. He put them on the plane and sadly never saw them again. He was killed by the Khmer Rouge after a few days.

Altogether we had twenty-four babies and small children to care for on that flight. At least two of them were really ill and receiving intravenous treatment. The rest needed frequent feeding and cried non-stop. The toddlers were very demanding and frightened. We recruited all the adults on board to be nurses and proxy parents. We had strapped down all the baskets to the plane floor and now we moved from cot to cot, checking, feeding, changing and comforting – what a job we had, with the plane taking off and making a short run to Bangkok. As we neared safety again, I rather gave out. I was emotionally totally drained and very concerned for all these young lives that were now my responsibility.

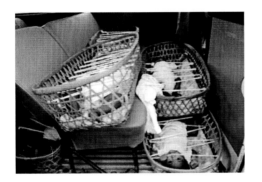

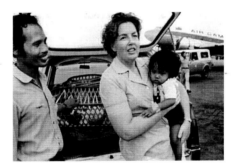

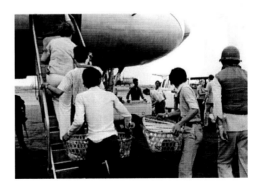

*Evacuating orphans by aeroplane, 12 April 1975*

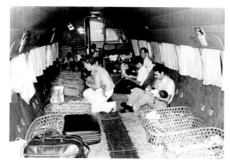

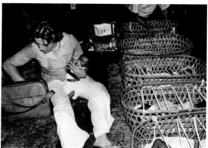

*Babies strapped down on the flight*

*Feeding in flight*

It was a hectic journey for Margaret and me, darting from one baby to the next. We got all our team feeding babies on the floor – they were rather good at it too. We made it safely and I sent up prayers of thanks. I really had not expected to see Bangkok again that day. We faced the same visa problems for our planeload of infants. They were allowed in as long as we promised to take them out again within one week. Our back-up Thailand team had been working hard to find a home for the babies on arrival, and we and they were welcomed into the large residence of an American lady, who even had cots organised. We handed them over to a team of volunteers, both Thai and expatriate. We took the sickest babies to a Thai hospital, where they were admitted and given expert care. I knew the one-week deadline would be impossible for these children, although most others could have travelled on immediately – but where to? I was not aware then that our two directors had been active for some time in anticipation that homes would be needed for young children.

We were soon told that World Vision International had arranged homes for twenty infants in prospective adoptee families in USA. It was all under the umbrella of an adoption agency in Los Angeles. I was not very happy about this, but had no better suggestion. All I could do was ensure the children were healthy for their long trip and wave them on their way after three days in Bangkok. It was hard to see them go, more especially because Margaret moved on home to Australia at the same time. Only I was left to sort out care for the hospitalised babies. All was well with two of them, who were sent home and ready to travel with the other children with a volunteer escort. I was left with a tiny, malnourished and very ill six-month baby called Phalla, far too ill to fly anywhere.

Then the Thai immigration officials started to press me: they wanted that baby out. I knew I could not take the child all the way across the ocean to east coast USA. She might well die en route. So I tried to find a country along the way where we could stop over. I opted for Hong Kong and found World Vision friends who would put us up. Of course I would go too. I had a British passport and therefore no problem getting into Hong Kong. I risked it with the child and no papers for her. In the event, when we got to Hong Kong immigration, they were not as helpful as I had hoped, the baby being so obviously ill. They agreed to a 48-hour stopover for both of us, and I went thankfully to our refuge house. They were very good to us and the baby settled down and even improved a little, so I decided to chance the long journey to Los Angeles. Once the crew knew I was a doctor, I was allowed on board with her. I prepared an intravenous line in place and infusion of sugar/saline – I could not risk more dehydration than she already had. So I laid her out on our two seats and sat with her lying across me.

The journey was a long one, but we made it. I had been assured we would be met and looked after. I was very tired myself. As we drew near to Los Angeles, I got messages through the captain that Stan Mooneyham himself would be there to meet us, along with the US media in force. I had no idea then the amount of media interest in these children. I soon learnt! I was to have the baby ready to be photographed on arrival. It wasn't hard to make her look starved and ill – she was. I handed her over to Stan at the aircraft door, sincerely hoping she would not vomit or have diarrhoea on him. I kept a very close watch on her and intervened as soon as I felt she had had enough of this public treatment. I escorted her to a children's hospital, where she received wonderful care and from where she was adopted, as far as I know. I know nothing of her life thereafter, but would love to know how she did.


## Civilisation again

I myself was welcomed into the World Vision family. I slept a good deal but also tried to help with the settling-in process for all the children. Adoptive parents needed to know much more about the medical history of each child and anything about their background that I knew: who was father? and mother? What was their fate? Most of all, I wanted to know what was happening to my dear friends and colleagues left behind. News from Cambodia was all bad; there was not much and anything there was caused distress. The main story was about the group of remaining expatriates who were detained in the French Embassy compound and eventually sent out to Thailand overland in trucks. I think I would have been on those trucks if I had stayed. Once they arrived, they told us all about the horrific city evacuation and the murder of most officials and educated Cambodians. I could not cope at all then, and needed support. I felt very alone and sensed that nobody understood.

*W V medical team 1974*

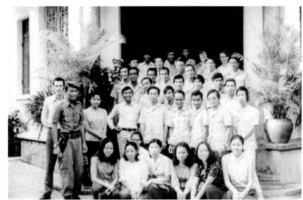

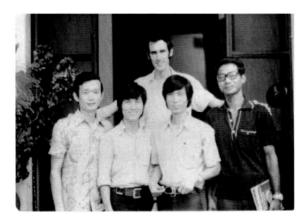

*An Australian colleague, Lindsay Nicholls, with four Cambodians, early 1975*

*A note here may be worthwhile: whereas I later realised that people in the UK had little or no interest in what had been happening in Cambodia, the people of the United States had a very different outlook. They had been so hugely involved over the war in Vietnam, and had seen the recent fall of that country, that they were very much concerned with what was going on in that part of the world at that time.*

***

## In a dark tunnel

My colleagues at World Vision (or wives of colleagues) took me on some 'cheer-up' outings. It was very kind of them, but I did not smile and laugh as they had hoped. Their first outing for me was Disneyland outside Los Angeles. I found it very difficult; all this luxury and fun – at what a price? When my children and dear friends across the world were dying of starvation and war!

I decided to go home to England and find something normal again. So off I flew to London and home. I know my parents were happy to see me, though I wasn't mentally in a good state. Today I would be labelled as a case of 'post-traumatic stress syndrome', but it had not been invented then. Looking back now, I know that I slept badly, had bad dreams and was very emotional.

What I found hardest was the seeming indifference of governments of the West to what was clearly happening. Why could we Western powers not intervene – with our military might? My old friends knew nothing about Cambodia and were not very interested to hear from me, and of course I had lost contact with Margaret and all the others who had shared the recent traumatic experiences with me. What was I to do next? Clearly, I could not return now. My main problem was that I had no money and certainly my parents could not afford to keep me for more than a few weeks. World Vision had not been generous to our team. We were sent away with one month's notice and one month's pay – the pay was not high anyway.

***

I had to earn money. So I started to scan the medical journals to find something that fitted my skills. It was not easy and I soon looked overseas again, to people's horror and disapproval. At home, I could have re-entered general practitioner training, but would have to go back to the beginning, which did not suit me. Careerwise, I had to decide whether to take up public health, which was becoming my obsession. Without funds, I could not afford the training I needed, so I decided to earn it somewhere and then train. So I had to seek a well-paid job – somewhere – that I was qualified to do. I soon found this meant somewhere overseas and I was rather glad, though most positions were not well paid.

My eye was caught by an advertisement for a well-paid job with a French mining company stationed in Zaïre (now DRC, the Democratic Republic of the Congo). They wanted a doctor with overseas and maternity experience to treat the wives and families of African and expatriate miners, and to live in a caravan on the mine's camp. One criterion was to be French-speaking. I applied and was invited to an interview to be conducted in French – gosh! was my French that good now? It turned out they only wanted someone who could converse with the French-speaking wives of staff about their medical problems. I had no difficulty at that level so soon found myself with a new adventure to take my mind off what was happening in Cambodia.

# Chapter 6: Africa 1975-78

## Zaïre 1975

I embarked again, this time for Africa, still very sad about Cambodia but glad to be working again in a familiar environment. The big difference was the Zaïrian people (the Zaïroise). They were living under a brutal military regime (Mobutu), and were hostile to expatriates. The mine and camp were in south east Zaïre, close to the Zambia border which we crossed frequently to get away from Zaïre and its problems.

The miners were an oppressed group of men from far and wide. They were not well paid, but for them *any* money was good pay. Most of them had large families – sometimes three or more wives and many children – to support. I got into trouble very early because of this. It was a strict rule of the company that medical treatment could only be provided to one wife and her children – not to any other children. As there was a measles epidemic when I arrived, I found this rule impossible to keep; I could not deny any of the sick little mites and used to lay them in rows on beds in the Cambodia way. This was appreciated by the men and women, but not by the company, who made it clear that I must conform. As they were fairly desperate for the medical help that I could offer, they just told me off and left it at that, and I called their bluff a few times.

There were two small clinics – one for expatriates and another, a mile or so away, for 'natives'. I had to travel between the two, which was hard at night, when the Zaïrian soldiers prowled around looking for likely victims, mostly from among the expats, whose vehicles they could drain of petrol. They were most unhelpful and I used to get angry with them – to no avail. But it worried me a lot when a young Frenchman received a severe beating one night and ended up on our doorstep half dead from a beating by soldiers. So I tried to get a driver and escort. The mine management failed to understand the need for night calls or visits to the native clinic, in the same way that they appeared content to allow women and young children to go untreated because they were not Number One wife or family.

# From Zaïre to Transkei

I had accepted a six-month contract with the mining company and agreed to extend for another three months while I decided what to do next. By this time I had saved enough money to broaden my choices. I wanted to continue in Africa and see more of it, and particularly to understand apartheid. I was not impressed with Zaïre – the people were so oppressed. I looked around again through the medical journals and found an advertisement for the United Society for the Propagation of the Gospel (USPG). They were looking for a doctor to be medical superintendent of an ex-Mission hospital in Transkei, a South Africa 'homeland'. I would be employed and paid by the Government of South Africa. I applied and was contacted very quickly and asked to take the post. I was on my way – and not very sorry to be leaving the copper mines, nor indeed to be leaving Zaïre. In the nine months of my time there, I had not even begun to integrate or to make enduring relationships with anyone from any of the communities: the local people, the French mining management or the immigrant work force. The medical team, itself mostly English like me, or Irish, were all very temporary.

## Transkei – The hospital and work

All Saints' Hospital was situated in the village of Engcobo in western Transkei, not far from East London. I flew to East London from Zaïre and was duly met by the retiring missionaries, the Ingles. Dr Pauline Ingle, who was originally English and by now in her late sixties, was a legend. She had run that hospital for some time, and had married an English surgeon, Ronald Ingle, after which they both continued there very happily for years, much loved by the staff and people they served. It was not easy to follow them – partly because I think they did not really want to leave and certainly had no confidence that I could manage when they left. It was a somewhat stormy handover.

All Saints' Hospital had been there as an Anglican mission hospital for many years. It had grown gradually in an unplanned way and was spread over a large area of land, with wards far from each other. The newest building was the operating theatre – purpose-built and comparatively modern. After my experiences in PNG I found the working conditions quite good. I was allocated a staff house to myself; it was quite large for one person, and I rather rattled around. All staff quarters there had servants' quarters attached, where a maid-cum-cook-housekeeper moved with her family into what I felt was very inadequate accommodation – but she was glad of it.

There were two young British doctors working with me at All Saints'. Tim and Sally Reynolds were good friends and helped settle me into a very demanding and different life and work regime. The local nurses were wonderful; they were mostly Christian, for although the hospital was now run by the government, the mission ethos prevailed. I could rely totally on the staff throughout the hospital – whether Matron, paediatric sister or senior midwife. They all knew their jobs totally and were committed to their patients. They were tolerant of us doctors, though often knew more than we did.

The hospital was large and very busy – a referral centre for a large district of about 200,000 people in a poor part of Transkei. Officially, there were 320 beds. But this was expandable by floor beds. The biggest job for the three of us, as medical officers, was daily outpatients. We saw several hundred, as well as coping with several accidents and emergencies every day. Many were simple breaks, lacerations and abscesses, but they all had to have treatment, sometimes in theatre. We had no surgeon then, though Tim did a good job as far as he could. I remember sometimes finishing after seven in the evening – and *still* having to do a round in 'my' wards, which were maternity, gynaecology and paediatrics.

## Road Accident – In charge again

Soon after I arrived, there was a tragic accident to my nursing staff, which not only left a deep impression on me, but also helped me to get the confidence of the local staff and people.

There was a strong South African Nursing Association and there were meetings at different hospitals most weekends. One fateful Saturday, I authorised most of the off-duty sisters, including the Matron, to travel to a sister mission hospital down near the sea for a meeting. They hired a minibus and set off early.

At about three o'clock in the afternoon, I received an emergency call from the host hospital to say that something dreadful had happened. Communications were very difficult but the police were on the scene and they came to me to tell me that through their radio network they had been notified of a serious accident on the very dangerous road down to the coast, and that it was my nursing sisters who had borne the brunt of the accident. Apparently, the minibus had lost control and plummeted over the side of the road and down a ravine. They thought there were deaths at the scene, but that most of the passengers had been taken to the local hospital. The staff left behind at All Saints' got together quickly to pray and then we had to notify the families. After another hour, I received a very frightened phone call from one of the paediatric sisters who had been on the bus. She told me what had happened, that most of the hospital sisters were now in hospital, and please would I send an ambulance to bring them back to All Saints'.

At once, I sent off a medical team with our ambulance to see what they could do. I did not go myself because I thought it better to get ready for them at home. Six of our sisters died that day. There were thirteen sisters on the bus, all senior, and only one was left able to walk; the other six had fractures to the pelvis and other injuries. All the injured came back and we put them into one of our wards all together. It was a very anxious time but every one survived, and most of them got back to work, but the loss of six staff was devastating to the hospital – and to me. Later, when I was talking to a senior government health officer about my first year, I remarked that it had been rather stressful and he asked why. I replied, 'Well, if thirteen of your staff had been involved in a very serious road accident and six killed, don't you think it would have been stressful?' He replied, 'I had forgotten that.'

I had to attend six funerals, and I learned that Transkei funerals were all-day events: there would have been an all-night wake the night before the day of the burial. Of course, this entailed my travelling out to the six different villages but fortunately I had a driver, and many from the hospital staff went too. I had to meet six different grieving families, making a speech on each occasion to people who very often had not themselves had further education. It was hard; costly and emotionally exhausting so soon after my arrival in the area, and there was still a hospital to run, but I was certainly bound to the community from this time on. Whereas I would have expected to get something back from the people in the way of a richer relationship, I did not really find it and the reason for that was apartheid.

I was very sad that I did not seem able to get close to senior African staff. In both Papua and Cambodia, my staff had become close friends but in the Transkei it was different. Although I worked closely with African doctors and nurses, it was always at arm's length. I was lonely and needed people to come home with me just to be sociable, but I could not persuade them to come. I was never invited to their houses and it was later explained to me. They said this was common: black Africans had no experience of entertaining white people because they had not ever been allowed to. And anyway, they did not think their houses were fit for white people, and they would not come to my house if I would not go to theirs. Of course I would have gone, but I was not made to feel welcome. They did gradually begin to come to mine on occasions, but in all my time there I was never able to break down this barrier.

I dealt with all the midwifery, which was challenging but interesting. I had to learn that the women of Transkei were far removed from Papuans as far as their pelvis was concerned: many had a condition of contracted pelvis, caused by childhood malnutrition, and I quickly saw my first, but by no means my last, ruptured uterus.

We treated many tuberculosis patients; it was the overriding medical condition there, often presenting in children as miliary TB, in which the whole body is affected, and the children were very ill and mostly died. There was a national TB programme in place, and we pioneered home treatment and followed up hundreds of patients in their villages, taking treatment at home. This has grown into the WHO's global programme of home treatment by supervised, long-term, oral drug therapy. There was a nearby 300-bed TB and leprosy hospital, which I and my small medical staff looked after. I used to spend one day a week there doing ward rounds; here my previous experience at St Luke's TB hospital in Papua stood me in good stead. Leprosy was an endemic disease, with many new cases identified each month out in remote villages.  Modern drug treatment had just been introduced but the chronic cases were beyond recovery, especially the deformities.

## Steve Biko – martyr

This great Transkei son died a martyr's death in police custody while I was working at All Saints'.  His estranged wife worked as a midwife in the maternity ward.  One tragic night it fell to me to tell her of her husband's death.  They had separated and she cared for their children.  Steve's parents and family lived in a suburb of Port Elizabeth, not so far away, but firmly in South African territory, where apartheid ruled.  As usual, I took no notice as I arranged to drive Steve's wife personally to his home in a black township, definitely out of bounds to whites, but I do remember feeling rather anxious, not knowing what reception I might get as a white woman from 'the enemy', responsible for Steve's untimely death.  I need not have worried.  When I walked into his house, his parents and brothers welcomed me graciously, thanked me profusely and fed me before I left.  There was no feeling of resentment or blame shown to me.  It was amazing.  But next day, back at All Saints', the hospital manager came to me rather shamefaced and said I needed to know that we had taken on two new members of staff that day.  I was surprised, as normally I would have a say in all appointments.  There were lots of winks and nods around until I was made to understand the true nature of these extras.  They were sent from South Africa to report on me personally.  My journey had not gone unnoticed by the South African police and now I was under scrutiny as a potential saboteur of apartheid.  But nothing further happened to me and after a while they melted into the background and finally disappeared.

## Night scare

It would be wrong to give the impression that we had no disorder problems. We were living in an area where white settlers had lived for probably at least five generations, and throughout the region there were lots of black villages dotted about. These were not enclosed and the situation was different from South Africa, but there was much violence and bitterness towards the white perpetrators of apartheid, especially the Afrikaners, around these villages where I often held clinics. I was mostly alone in my house at night, although my maid lived in her quarters at the back. It could be quite scary, especially when I was called to the hospital for night emergencies, a common occurrence. And although there was a hospital night watchman, he did not cover staff quarters, so I was anxious much of the time.

One particular night I vividly remember waking suddenly, knowing there was someone else in the room. By the moonlight I could make out the shadow of a black man standing over me as I lay in bed. He seemed to be holding something ready to strike me. I tried to call out, but no sound came. However, as I moved around and leapt to my feet, he ran off. I never found what he took, if anything. I have a feeling that the staff did not believe me next morning, mainly as there was nothing to show for the intrusion. This was the second time in my life overseas that I had unwelcome visitors at night. The first had been while working in Port Moresby, where I had repelled burglars late one night. They were caught. My big problem was that I could not with certainty identify the men later; black faces at night are very black and features are hard to make out. Does one just say, 'Yes, that was him,' when unsure? It's hardly right. Anyway, my Transkei intruder was never found.


## Surprise

I was distracted late one evening just after my first Christmas in Transkei by a sudden phone call from the Foreign Office in London. I was told by a stranger that I had been recognised in the Queen's New Year Honours List for my work in Cambodia. This came completely out of the blue; I had not thought of such a thing, and now I was asked if I would accept an OBE. My first thought was how proud my parents would be. I could not refuse. I realised I had to telephone Dad at once or they would read it in the papers before I told them. I did so, and although they knew, they did not let on. I never knew if it was leaked to them, but I suspect it was. Of course, they were thrilled.

***

I went home in June of that year (1977), to receive my honour at Buckingham Palace from the Queen. My parents came with me and my brother John chauffeured us to the Palace. After the ceremony, my parents threw a party for me at their London club. Many dear friends attended but sadly no one from my team in Cambodia – there simply wasn't anyone in the UK. Nevertheless, it was a very great occasion in my life.

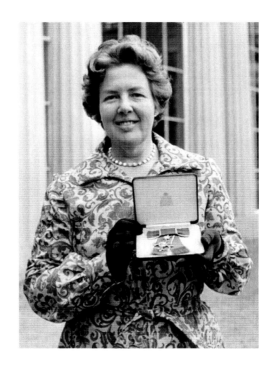

*With my OBE*

## And back in Transkei

After my first year in South Africa, following my home visit and with no prospect of more medical staff, I was suffering seriously from work overload. Maternity was my biggest headache and it drained me more every day. Patient numbers rose dramatically as we became well known for our success with mothers and babies. My midwife sister used to say, 'You are getting well known and all the women try to come here now.' Many came to wait to have their babies with us and we set up a maternity waiting shelter for just this purpose. The hospital was overflowing with floor beds. But this flood from outside did not detract from the regular load of deliveries and emergency admissions we were already dealing with.

I had become experienced at dealing with the many difficulties suffered by the women of this poor region, where young women had been undernourished since early childhood and were very often chronically anaemic. I delivered many infants by Caesarean section. I had been very unhappy both giving an anaesthetic and conducting the operation concurrently, and while in London, I had learned the technique of epidural injection. Early on, I introduced the use of epidural anaesthesia for all my C-sections. I suspect the Transkei women, as well as the staff, thought I was practising magic, when I injected in their backs and delivered their babies painlessly while they stayed awake. The staff took a lot of convincing, but I knew all was well when the senior maternity sister opted for an epidural to deliver her third child. It certainly saved lots of problems from sleepy babies – often the result of heavy ether anaesthetic. Our babies came out screaming and well. Our maternity statistics were excellent, but not so our general paediatric results. There, the common conditions we struggled against included mastoiditis, osteomyelitis, TB, anaemia, and malnutrition with kwashiorkor, and the mortality was high.

## Medical students

These were the years when UK medical schools encouraged final year medical students to spend a year or so in a developing country to gain practical experience. These students could be very useful to the places where they were posted, but with one proviso. Existing medical staff had to spend time teaching them and then supervising them. It was not fair to them to expect them just to be workhorses, with no gain to themselves, as they were not paid – just provided with food and accommodation.

At All Saints' I was lucky that a link had already been established with a

London medical school (St Barts). This meant we were on a list of places for students to go for good experience. They usually came in twos or more. We took up to six if possible. We had some excellent students, who helped us hugely, and I'm sure they gained from what we taught them. Their first responsibility was usually in the casualty department, where they examined and diagnosed patients, arranged X-rays and laboratory tests and then referred the patient to one of us doctors for treatment. After a short time, most students were allowed to go ahead and start treatment for many cases, especially simple trauma and broken limbs. If they were good enough I then liked to teach them to administer a simple anaesthetic, so that they could undertake minor operations by themselves. If they showed great aptitude, then they were allowed to concentrate on developing that particular skill. I remember several that used to give general anaesthetics in theatre for quite major operations. After all, none of us was a trained anaesthetist, so they could easily be as good (or bad) as we were!

I remember teaching several students to give spinal and epidural anaesthetic for operations, especially to assist me in theatre with Caesarean sections, where I was usually both giving anaesthetic and doing the surgery, so their help was most valuable and I was always very sorry to see a student leave to go and take the dreaded final exams. I feel sure they were better doctors from what they learned with me and my other staff, including the nursing staff. I wish I knew where they are now.

Then, there was always the tiresome time of welcoming a new batch of students, assessing their capacity and starting them to work – teaching all the time; but it was worth it for the several months' return when they performed as good house officers and junior doctors.

\*\*\*

Our scarce medical staff was on call all the time. I was very tired, getting up most nights for maternity cases. I think I was pretty impossible to work with – but it was tiredness. I realised that something had to give and in the end it was me. I asked for early leave and went to stay with South African friends to rest. There I thought long and hard about my future, realising that things were not likely to get any better at All Saints'. I could see then that this was not the place to spend the rest of my life and I was sure that God had something else for me. At this time I still had my Cambodian team and friends much on my mind and in my heart. News was filtering out by now of atrocities and killings in Cambodia. Indeed, two survivors of my medical team there had contacted me one way or another (I wish we had had e-mail then). I had received a phone call from a refugee camp in Vietnam from Dr Sokphan. He told me of his escape from Cambodia with his family and his hard life now in a re-education camp in Saigon. He asked me to help him get a visa for France or the UK. I was too far away and too poor to help him, though I was thrilled to hear from him. He did not have good news of the rest of our team and I was devastated, especially by the deaths of Dr Kim Nguon and Dr Mam Bun Thol.

Next I had news from World Vision that my dear friend Kanyaket (Kan) had emerged from exile, but was ill with malnutrition and probable TB. I could offer little help and could only send money and ask World Vision to help her get treatment. I wondered how best I could do more to help the family. I believe this is what led me to realise it was time to get a proper 'earning job' so that I had at least some money available for the urgent needs of my friends. My pay in Transkei was not too bad except that we were then not allowed to take any South African currency out of the country, so saving was not productive.

***

When I look back now, although I was not happy during the time I have just written about, I suppose my African experience was an interlude which fulfilled an immediate need. I went there because I wanted to know what apartheid was, wanting to learn about it, and I came to understand the enormous needs and problems of Africa. It helped me in the rest of my life, especially my time in London, when I needed a global orientation, not a focus on just one area.

# Chapter 7: Back to the UK and away again: Overseas Development Administration 1978-82

As always, God had an answer. I was scanning every paper I could get hold of and all the medical journals – there was no internet then – for suitable jobs. I felt I needed to study more: I was only 39, rising 40, and my rather basic qualifications did not impress UK employers. I thought I would be best suited to general practice, although even for that I would need to take more courses and exams. But, as so often, my brother John came to my rescue. He found and sent me a job advert for a position as Overseas Development Health Advisor to the British Government: a well-paid civil service appointment. (The ODA later became the Department for International Development – or DFID.) The lights were all green, not red, and so I applied from my present job and even lined up the money for an airfare if I was lucky enough to get an interview. Of course, I had to give in my notice and as a result I had an interview with the new Transkei Health Minister and was offered a transfer to another Transkei hospital. I was tempted but did not accept; I think I said that if my London application was not successful, I might reconsider – I could not afford to be unemployed. I went home to my excited, now elderly, parents, who thought I would now settle down at home. Little did they know!

I was not really hopeful of the job – what did I know of governments and aid programmes? I had worked mainly on the 'other side' for NGOs and was hardly tolerant of what governments did or did not do. I think I told them that at the interview. I know the other candidates were all men and well known to the ODA. I was the only woman short-listed and this was to my advantage as time was ripe for women to be sought for senior posts in the civil service. Some would say we were given an unfair advantage. I did not agree then. I was still agonising over the right path to go down and I had job interviews lined up for a general practice position. I was told I would be contacted about the result of the ODA interview in a few days – at most, a week. But I also had a deadline for the GP job, being told emphatically not to present myself if I had any doubts. So I was in a fix, waiting to hear if I had the ODA job, which by now I really wanted. I cheekily rang the ODA, refusing to wait patiently. It was as well I did. A very sympathetic woman told me that I was to be offered the job, starting as soon as I was available. So I turned down the GP interview and accepted the ODA post with excited anticipation. The family were delighted.

***

My first task was to find somewhere to live in London. I was totally inexperienced in urban living – in the UK or anywhere else. My advantage was that my youngest brother, Rob, had now married and was teaching at Harrow School. He and his wife Sue took pity on me and gave me a room and board on a temporary basis until I could find my own place. I loved getting to know them again and their small children, Adam and Sophy; Helen soon came along too, and became my much-loved goddaughter. Rob helped me to house-hunt and I soon was able to take out my first mortgage and buy a one-bedroom flat in Kennington, very near my ODA office in Victoria. But I am jumping ahead of my adaptation to my very new and different job.

## The ODA London, 1978

This new job presented me with the most enormous challenge. It was totally different from any other job I had ever done, but was fulfilling my dream to become a public health expert. I had no patients and could no longer claim to my disgusted nephews and nieces to be a 'proper doctor'. They could not understand how anyone could be a doctor and not treat patients! I had to accept that I now had a desk job; no night calls, and free evenings and nights. I still worked very hard, doing many extra hours at the office, and I spent hours reading files – and then there was the travel. When I started at ODA, I was the Assistant Medical Advisor, working for two senior advisors, who undertook to teach me and shepherd me round my first overseas assignment. I already knew that they did not approve of, or like having, a woman advisor. There had not been one before at ODA. As in several previous jobs, I weathered the prejudice and proved, I think, that I could do it as well as they could. Sometimes there were storms in the corridors. I was encouraged along the way by my wise friend, Barbara, the Nursing Advisor, who faced the same issues regularly, and naturally we teamed up.

To explain the job: we were each individually allocated a part of the world or a country and were billed in the office directory as medical advisor for that place. This meant that all health or medical queries about 'my' countries were routed to me to answer – all from the dreaded files. Most of the questions related to the health services of that country and how the ODA could help it to develop or improve the service: for example, by providing a new hospital, laboratories, a pharmacy, etc. More interesting was the assistance that could be given to developing countries and providing staff for their health service. The Caribbean Commonwealth islands, including Antigua, St Kitts and Nevis, St Lucia, Grenada and Anguilla, were assigned to me. I visited most of them every year and learned that sun, sand and blue sky was not the whole picture. There was a lot of poverty for the inhabitants and a lack of good training establishments. I enjoyed my visits to the University of the West Indies in Jamaica and the Caribbean Epidemiology Centre in Trinidad, both doing excellent training work for nearby countries and providing consultancies for their essential health services.

In its previous life as the Colonial Office, the Overseas Development Ministry (the ODM, now the ODA – Administration), had traditionally provided many doctors, nurses and paramedical staff for hospitals all round the world. There was a much-loved scheme called OSAS (Overseas Supplement Aid Scheme) which recruited senior health or medical staff in Britain to fill vacancies in a country's health establishment, e.g. surgeons, paediatricians and gynaecologists. These people were seconded to the overseas government and paid a local salary, but this rather low salary was then augmented considerably by the ODA up to the level they would expect if they worked in the British NHS. It was my job to find and recruit these people, to refer them to the overseas country concerned, brief the outgoing specialist and even work out what they should be paid. Some of these medicos did extremely well for themselves and led a very pleasant life overseas.

At first I felt privileged to be visiting these exotic and beautiful places, but they were like nowhere else I had been before. They were not really 'third world'. The people were educated and often well trained in many professions; they had well-trained teachers and nurses and were making great strides in training doctors and medical specialists, but the islands were poor and governments not able to pay their public servants well, so many professionals left the islands for a better life in Canada, the US or the UK, where they were welcomed for their skills and were more satisfied with their standard of living. Tourism was the major industry and groups of islands, like the British Virgin Isles and the Turks and Caicos Islands, were famous throughout North America. How beautiful they were and how I loved them, though they were not easy to help through our Aid Programme, which was more targeted to the needs of the least developed countries and primary health care services than to developing hospitals in the previous colonies.

Another interesting experience I gained then was representing the British Dependencies at the annual meetings of the Pan-American Health Organisation (PAHO) in Washington, DC. I began to learn and understand the workings of the World Health Organisation, which stood me in good stead in my future work. I enjoyed going to Washington almost every year for a while, in the 1980s, usually coinciding with visits to the Caribbean islands – colonies or previous colonies. I was privileged to be there several years when these previous colonies had become independent from Britain and were welcomed into PAHO as full members in their own right (not just represented by Britain). But I continued to represent the interests of Bermuda, the Cayman Islands, the British Virgin Islands, the Turks and Caicos Islands, Anguilla and Montserrat.

It was very interesting to meet the Health Ministers and officials from the South American countries: Mexico, Peru and others. I had an interesting encounter with the Argentinean delegation the year of the Falkland Islands conflict (*Islas Malvinas* to them). I found myself in a minibus on my own with some ten Argentineans. At first I felt threatened but in the end we all saw the funny side and behaved as health colleagues.

I learned then how to speak my mind in a large conference setting and how best to use interpreters; there were a lot of Spanish-speaking countries in the Americas. I was not a silent delegate and sometimes challenged the organisation if I thought it was wrong or unfair. I was becoming known as a champion of women's participation and rights, and one year I remember the PAHO officials proudly presenting statistics for all the training scholarships

151

they had awarded to member-states over the last several years. I at once intervened to request a breakdown by gender. To their huge embarrassment, officials finally admitted a serious under-representation of women among these trainees – almost none! But PAHO women staff cheered me on (to my own embarrassment now) and asked me to take up their cause to obtain more training and better conditions (especially equal pay) for women staff. On one occasion, the woman interpreter translating my English into Spanish (for the Latins) went outside her remit and cheered me on, strongly endorsing what I said. I'm afraid I became a thorn in the flesh for the Regional Director and his staff but, in retrospect, I was right.

***

During those years I travelled to many poor countries on behalf of the British Government: for example, Bolivia, Honduras, Belize, the Falkland Islands, Pakistan, Bangladesh, and the Pacific islands of the Solomons, Vanuatu and Kiribati. Incidents from this time that I remember particularly include the following from Bolivia, Pakistan, the Falkland Islands and Vanuatu.

## Bolivia

The ODA had agreed to support one remote district in Bolivia to develop a primary health care service through renovating and establishing rural health services and training village health workers. I was tasked with visiting the district to monitor progress and agree the next stages with Bolivian health staff. I flew through the mountains to La Paz and landed at the very high-altitude airport, where just stepping out of the plane and walking to the lounge made one breathless. It took me several days to acclimatise so that I could work. On my first day I called at the Embassy, where our Ambassador had an office on the second floor of an old building. Most of his visitors must have been very breathless when they reached him! I stayed at a modest hotel in La Paz and was puzzled to receive callers my second day; they were tin mine workers who had somehow found out that there was a British woman staying at the hotel. They invited me to go to a meeting they had called nearby, as people wanted me to take a message back to Britain. It was all about pay and conditions in their mines. They felt badly treated and underpaid and wanted the British people to know and help them. Such a thing had never happened to me before and I was interested but knew I could do little to help them. All I could do (and did) was to tell our Ambassador about it and leave it to our local representatives to advise.

## Project visit: Sucré

Then it was 'project' time. Our small team flew off through the high mountains to a district town – Sucré – where we met with doctors and public health officials to discuss the work and see clinics. From the town we drove a long way on appalling roads out to health centres in villages. We were always met by crowds of people, all grateful for our work. Our last visit involved me making a long trek on foot up a river bed – about three hours' walk – to reach a remote new health centre. The countryside was some of the most inhospitable I had ever encountered. There was no water, but arid dry soil with stones underfoot, with women and children trying to scratch a living by growing potatoes. The women had to dig down several feet to reach just a little muddy water and then to carry it in a gourd to their house or to the plants. I remember being very thirsty and hot and finally puffing up a hill to reach the new heath centre, where many people were waiting to celebrate our visit. I was given a bucket with liquid in it. I did not know what it was, but the doctors and nurses all nodded encouragement for me to drink it, so I did, enthusiastically, although it tasted awful. Then they told me it was their local beer, made from fermenting potatoes and maize. Certainly, it was alcoholic and I felt good for a while, until it caught up with me. What a beautiful country it was, but how poor! And how hard their life was. Both infant and maternal mortality rates were among the highest in the world. I hope our input made some difference.

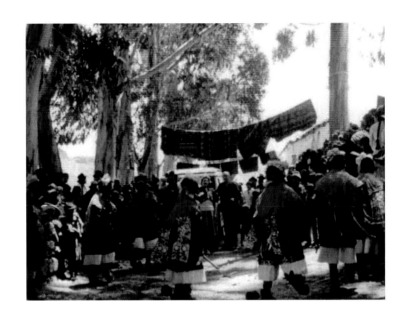

*Greeting at Puerta Sucré*

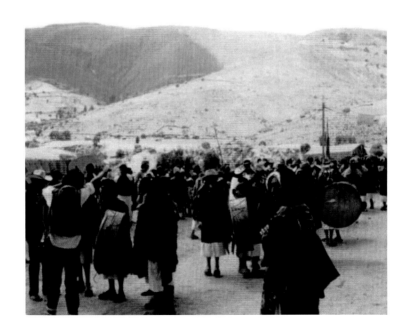

*Gathering for a celebration*

154

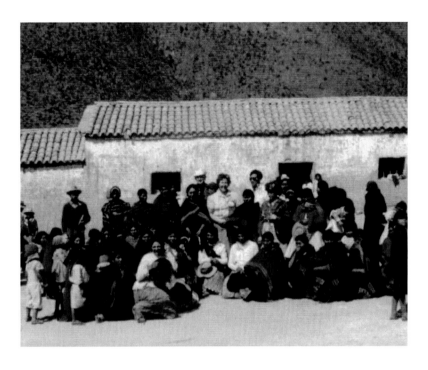

*A village group at San Jacinto*

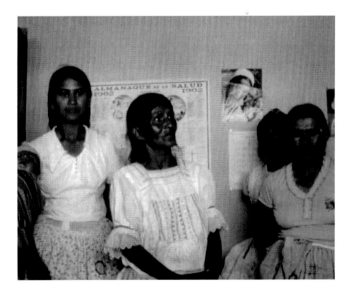

*Sotomajor – village health promoters*

# Pakistan, 1982

The British aid programme worked closely with many voluntary organisations (NGOs), like Save the Children, Oxfam and others. There was a special drive for us to partner and fund NGOs which were based in the developing countries themselves and where most of the staff were nationals of the country. One such organisation was the Aga Khan Foundation, with education and health projects throughout Pakistan. I was delighted to have an opportunity to visit one health project in northern Pakistan, close to the Afghan border. Our small team started work at the HQ in Peshawar, where we joined a large team of Pakistani health and education senior staff – all men. I was mortified my first evening to be relegated to a table by myself for dinner and was angry at being deserted by my (male) ODA colleagues, who I had thought would have been sensitive to such discrimination. But the trip was worth it. Next day we set off in small army helicopters, following the ancient silk route up to the northern states. We crossed the very high mountains, quite short of oxygen and too close to the summits for comfort. We landed in the snow in Chitral for a community meeting to discuss health care with the village leaders (all men). I was detailed off from the meeting to go and talk to the nurses and some women they had lined up, including village health workers and birth attendants. I had a fascinating time and learned a lot about living as a woman in these harsh conditions. By this time, I was well wrapped up in a suitable headscarf, partly to seem respectable to the men, but also to keep warm.

That was my first visit to Pakistan but not my last. Another time I was taken to the North West Frontier Province to work with government health officials being supported by the ODA. I was taken by jeep to the old frontier towns, famous from stories of the frontier wars. The whole area was strongly defended and we were warned most emphatically against showing ourselves outside the hospitals, where we were within range of Taliban rebel guns. I was taken to refugee camps of Afghan people, fleeing from the Taliban regime. Again, I found similarities to Cambodia scenes.

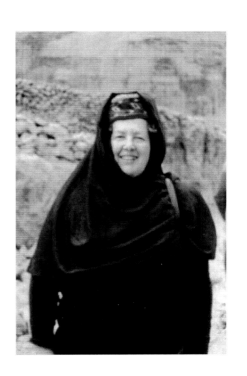

*Dressed for Chitral, Medical Advisor integrating for cultural acceptability*

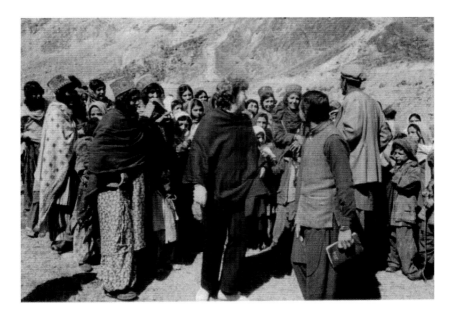

*Pakistan 1982, with a crowd of local people*

157

# The Falkland Islands

During the war of 1982, one young doctor, Alison Fury, funded by the ODA, did a marvellous job for which she was deservedly awarded an OBE. She ran the small hospital, liaised with and helped the British Army medical teams, and continued to care for the islanders throughout the war.

I was tasked with visiting her and planning with her and other officials the future health services. My question – how soon and how was I to go? Then Mrs Thatcher went out in an Air Force plane, so why not me? I pressured a bit. It was all arranged and I found myself, with our nursing advisor, at Brize Norton and thence en route to Ascension Island along with around 70 soldiers. There was nothing remarkable about that flight, other than sitting facing backwards in the plane. We landed on Ascension Island very late at night and disembarked under instruction to report at 0600 hours for the onward flight to Port Stanley. We were herded into a large army tent, where the men were detailed off into camp tents for the short night. They all left and we waited and wondered. I approached the sergeant in charge and said, 'What about us? Where shall we go?' He said with irritation, 'No one told us any women were coming, and there is no accommodation here for you. You will have to stay here in the tent for the night.' I was not impressed and suggested in a firm voice that he should try the nurses' quarters which I knew existed. We accepted with alacrity an invitation to go to the sister's house and stay there. I think we shared sofa-beds, but anything would have done. Next morning we were out at the airport for camp breakfast before flying. It was my first and last experience of a soldiers' camp breakfast – a big fry-up and not my favourite at that time.

After that large and greasy breakfast, we were all told to embark on the aeroplane. Sitting on the tarmac at Ascension Island (a vast airport on a tiny island) was a really old Hercules – propeller-driven, resembling what I had been used to in Papua. It was the only plane that could make the long distance and the runways either end, but needed refuelling mid-air on the way, a new phenomenon then. The men all climbed the short stairway and into the plane. I found myself nearly last on board and by this time (6.00 am) the pilots were shouting at us to hurry up. There were no seats to be seen. The men were all jammed together and sitting on canvas seats – just

158

pieces of webbing strung from the back to the front of the plane. A young officer took pity on me and made room for me next to him. This was greeted by much ribaldry from all the men nearby. We were strapped into place and the plane took off noisily. We were given earphones to muffle the engine noise. We were told to settle down for a 13-hour journey, which in this crowded plane was not going to be fun. There was no room to move around. I had no idea whether we would be given any food on the journey. However, my doubts were soon allayed when white lunch boxes were handed out to everybody, including me. By this time I was quite friendly with the officer at my side. He was kind and seemed to understand my predicament in a plane full of a hundred men. First he showed me how to put my feet up on the webbing opposite me. They had a system: as long as everyone put their feet on the opposite side then we were all jammed in safely and comfortably and at very close quarters. It was certainly very cosy, except that the noise level from the engines was very high.

But my next predicament had then to be faced. I could not see any sign of toilets and wondered what on earth to do. Along the side of the aeroplane there were urinals strategically placed. Of course, the men were too embarrassed to use them in my part of the plane. They had to cross over to the other side. I asked my officer what to do. He said, 'Oh, that's all right: you will have to climb along the webbing seat, over all the men to the back, where there is a private toilet, where canvas sides can be let down like a tent.' So eventually, I performed this gymnastic feat: I stood up on the seat and climbed over 20 or 30 men, who all obligingly jeered and cheered me on. Eventually, I reached the insubstantial tent-toilet. What a business it was! I think I went twice during the 13-hour journey and hung on for the rest. I asked the men how Mrs Thatcher had managed two weeks before? They quickly responded that she was all right as they had put a caravan into the Hercules for her journey, so she had it comfortable!

## Refuelling

The next excitement was when the plane was refuelled in mid-air. The captain told us that he would attempt to refuel at a certain time. If he were unsuccessful, he would need to land. The nearest landing possible was in

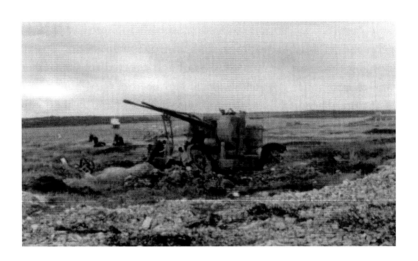

*Gun on the headland, trained on Argentina*

As well as the hospital, it was my job to understand the services and needs of the remote communities living on the outer islands. A visit was arranged and one early morning Alison and I climbed into a helicopter to be shown all round the islands. It was an amazing day, with wonderful views. We visited several of the cemeteries, still freshly dug and full of flowers. We landed at remote farm houses to meet local people and hear their needs. It was clear that the troops were making a huge difference at all levels. I was interested to look at their living conditions too. One farmer's wife told me proudly that soldiers came to her house once a week for a hot bath and to wash clothes. She was very good to them.

Then I met the Gurkha regiment, which was a thrill. They had made a huge contribution in the war and were camped in an inaccessible place where the only other inhabitants were sheep. The problem for the health staff was that the Gurkha soldiers used to slaughter sheep to eat. It had emerged that a disease called cysticercosis existed in the sheep on the Falklands – and was transferable to humans. So it was forbidden to slaughter and consume these sheep to prevent the nasty illness. But despite warnings, the Gurkhas would not comply. They really loved their mutton curry and especially a mutton spit-roast on a fire outside. They were highly resistant to giving up the meat. We all tried to convince them, but to no avail.

My fascinating tour of the outer islands ended dramatically. We hovered

162

pieces of webbing strung from the back to the front of the plane. A young officer took pity on me and made room for me next to him. This was greeted by much ribaldry from all the men nearby. We were strapped into place and the plane took off noisily. We were given earphones to muffle the engine noise. We were told to settle down for a 13-hour journey, which in this crowded plane was not going to be fun. There was no room to move around. I had no idea whether we would be given any food on the journey. However, my doubts were soon allayed when white lunch boxes were handed out to everybody, including me. By this time I was quite friendly with the officer at my side. He was kind and seemed to understand my predicament in a plane full of a hundred men. First he showed me how to put my feet up on the webbing opposite me. They had a system: as long as everyone put their feet on the opposite side then we were all jammed in safely and comfortably and at very close quarters. It was certainly very cosy, except that the noise level from the engines was very high.

But my next predicament had then to be faced. I could not see any sign of toilets and wondered what on earth to do. Along the side of the aeroplane there were urinals strategically placed. Of course, the men were too embarrassed to use them in my part of the plane. They had to cross over to the other side. I asked my officer what to do. He said, 'Oh, that's all right: you will have to climb along the webbing seat, over all the men to the back, where there is a private toilet, where canvas sides can be let down like a tent.' So eventually, I performed this gymnastic feat: I stood up on the seat and climbed over 20 or 30 men, who all obligingly jeered and cheered me on. Eventually, I reached the insubstantial tent-toilet. What a business it was! I think I went twice during the 13-hour journey and hung on for the rest. I asked the men how Mrs Thatcher had managed two weeks before? They quickly responded that she was all right as they had put a caravan into the Hercules for her journey, so she had it comfortable!

## Refuelling

The next excitement was when the plane was refuelled in mid-air. The captain told us that he would attempt to refuel at a certain time. If he were unsuccessful, he would need to land. The nearest landing possible was in

Brazil, but Brazil was not friendly to Britain at that time. Brazil supported Argentina in their claim for ownership of the Falkland Islands. So the captain was worried in case our plane was denied landing rights. There would not be enough fuel to get us back to Ascension Island. So the refuelling process was crucial for us. The captain invited my officer friend and me to go up to the flight deck to observe the refuelling. It was interesting and very exciting. A small plane came into sight alongside us, trailing a pipe with a cone attached to the back. They explained to me that they had to connect the nose of the Hercules into the cone to draw fuel down the pipe. We made two attempts that failed. On the final try, the captain was successful and we were all vastly relieved and cheered him loudly.

Our lunch proved to be an extraordinary collection of army rations. I was amazed how much food was in the box. There were the hard army biscuits that one expects. But as well as that, there were tins of baked beans, spam and potato salad. I looked rather helplessly at these tins and asked, 'How on earth will I open this?' Quite a few hands shot out offering to open them for me. There was a very small tin-opener buried in the box and the men had no trouble at all cutting open tins. I learned that, for lunch, a soldier was provided with 5,000 calories for his ration. After all this adventure, I could only eat a very small amount and gave the rest away to my willing neighbours.

At long last, after thirteen noisy hours, the lights of Port Stanley came into view. We landed at the army base, where the young doctor (Alison) I had come to visit met me. I was taken off to the only hotel and spent a night full of dreams about flying. I had still to make the return journey!

## Port Stanley Hospital

My main job was to report on the state of the main hospital in the Islands. As a British colony, our government was committed to employing sufficient qualified staff to meet the needs of the people. That meant doctors and senior nurses recruited in Britain and resident for a two-year appointment or longer. It required a very special medical skill to provide a good service without easy referral support to British specialists. There had to be a general surgeon and an anaesthetist, as well as someone with good midwifery skills. During the short war, army medical staff had covered for local emergencies as well as army ones. A field hospital had been opened but the army also used the main hospital – a pleasant, wooden structure by the seafront. It was adequate for the people's needs, but wanting some repairs and rehabilitation. I had good meetings with local people to hear their views. They were all very mindful of the war problems and risks they had faced in the last months – I know I was worried about safety aspects at the hospital: it was an old wooden structure and fire precautions were inadequate. Also there were a number of elderly residents occupying wards on a long-term basis, because of the breakdown in family structures with most young people leaving the Islands to work somewhere else. But I was unprepared and deeply shocked back home soon after my visit to hear that the hospital had been destroyed by fire one night, with some loss of life. Now there is a new and safer structure built.

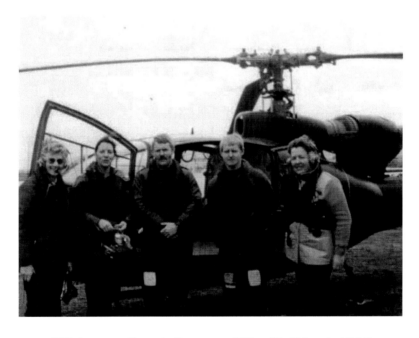

*With our valiant heli-crew on West Falkland, 1983*

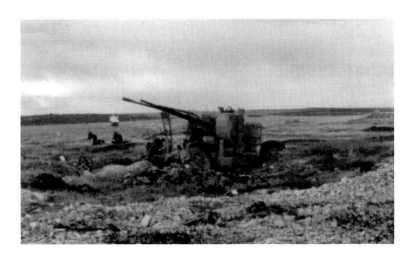

*Gun on the headland, trained on Argentina*

As well as the hospital, it was my job to understand the services and needs of the remote communities living on the outer islands. A visit was arranged and one early morning Alison and I climbed into a helicopter to be shown all round the islands. It was an amazing day, with wonderful views. We visited several of the cemeteries, still freshly dug and full of flowers. We landed at remote farm houses to meet local people and hear their needs. It was clear that the troops were making a huge difference at all levels. I was interested to look at their living conditions too. One farmer's wife told me proudly that soldiers came to her house once a week for a hot bath and to wash clothes. She was very good to them.

Then I met the Gurkha regiment, which was a thrill. They had made a huge contribution in the war and were camped in an inaccessible place where the only other inhabitants were sheep. The problem for the health staff was that the Gurkha soldiers used to slaughter sheep to eat. It had emerged that a disease called cysticercosis existed in the sheep on the Falklands – and was transferable to humans. So it was forbidden to slaughter and consume these sheep to prevent the nasty illness. But despite warnings, the Gurkhas would not comply. They really loved their mutton curry and especially a mutton spit-roast on a fire outside. They were highly resistant to giving up the meat. We all tried to convince them, but to no avail.

My fascinating tour of the outer islands ended dramatically. We hovered over a cliff with the sea just below us. Suddenly and without warning, our pilot landed and indicated that he was going to take off quickly. He pointed his hand inland and said, 'Go and see those people over there.' Alison and I got out quickly from the helicopter and set out across the heather and turf in the direction he had pointed. We could see nothing that indicated any people were there. We had a good look round and realised that there was a turret sticking up out of the ground on a small hillock. While we watched, a gun emerged and circled around, pointing mostly out to sea. We were amazed and quite scared. We went and had a good look and discovered a hole behind the gun and leading down somewhere. Now we could hear voices coming from below the ground. We shouted and a man answered us and then suddenly emerged from the hole. He was dressed in army uniform and did not seem fazed to see us. He told us that there were several more soldiers down the hole, and invited us in for a cup of tea. So down we went, giving a cheerful wave to the helicopter overhead. We just hoped it would come back for us. These six or eight men, all Welsh, gave us a great welcome, and we were able to find out a lot about their living conditions and their diet. It was not too bad. They considered themselves as look-outs. They kept the gun trained on Argentina in the far west. I couldn't help thinking to myself that we had managed to come into their hole without them knowing that we were close to them. Surely it would be just as easy for the enemy to creep up on them? Anyway, we eventually went up and found our helicopter waiting to land and take us back to Port Stanley. It had been a great day, though I'm almost sure it was a put-up job!

I stayed there for two weeks and it was fascinating. I was not looking forward to the journey home. However, in the end, the journey was not so bad, mainly because the plane was evacuating a number of injured men or sick people back to the UK, so there was an army medical team on board, including several nurses. I didn't feel quite so much on my own as on the journey out. We stopped at Ascension Island again and landed back at Brize Norton the next day. Then it was back to London to finish my report and try to persuade the ODA to provide some more funds for training health workers and for refurbishing the hospital. Unfortunately, my visit was not repeated, and now I understand that the Islands have plenty of money from fishing and can pay well for their own staff and health services.

# Vanuatu

I loved visiting the Pacific Islands. They were close to Papua where I started out on my career journey. Both the Solomon Islands and Vanuatu were peopled by Melanesians who spoke Pidgin – a little different from my Highlands Pidgin but similar enough to get by. At that time, Britain and Australia were providing sizeable assistance to the young nations, especially health and education services. Britain still provided a good number of senior medical staff and I had to visit them all and monitor their work. At the same time, it was my job to discuss all future assistance in the health sector, in line with ODA policies. Vanuatu was very similar, being the ex-Franco/British colony that had been called the New Hebrides. The ODA managed these programmes from Fiji, which gave me a great opportunity to visit that interesting place at a time of political turmoil after a coup in 1984.

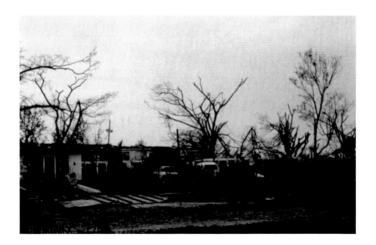

*After a cyclone in Vanuatu*

The Pacific has cyclones, as opposed to hurricanes, though they seem identical to me. In the cyclone season, one never knew if visits would be possible. If there was a cyclone warning, all planes were grounded, so no visits were possible. On one memorable visit to Port Vila, the capital of Vanuatu, a cyclone was forecast to hit the town the day I got there and I was put up in a very new but rather insubstantial hotel surrounded by coconut

164

trees. That night was one of the worst in my life. It was usual to stock up with candles, torches and buckets, but only those who had been through it before knew the wisdom of filling the bath with cold water and boarding up the picture windows, using beds standing on end. As the wind power increased, so the other hotel residents gathered in shock – mostly in my room. I suppose I was calmer than most and must have seemed confident. Two families with little children were terrified as the hotel roof blew off with a whoosh early in the night. Then the rain came down in sheets, and the roofless hotel rooms, with all their belongings, were soaked through. We all battened down in my bedroom, which was pretty wet, but holding out. We soon gave up the struggle of keeping the water out altogether; we coped with it as it came in, keeping everything possible off the floor, especially the two beds, where all the children were bedded down.

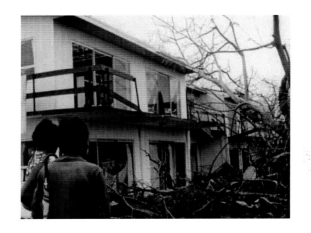

*The scene of our vigil: my bedroom underneath*

My room was under about two feet of dirty water. Of course, there were no lights so we felt cold, despite the tropical temperature. After a long time it grew quieter outside; the wind began to die down and we heard no more trees crashing down or roofs being torn off. It became a dark, wet, night. We all huddled together, grateful for company but not able to do anything useful until dawn came – in its usual fast way – and we were able to look around us. There was utter devastation to everything we could see: the hotel, the trees, the pool – my room. But we had come through unscathed.

165

The small children woke up fretful but quite well. We were all hungry. Among us all we produced some rations – biscuits and a little bread, but not enough for long. I had filled thermos flasks before the power went off, so I made hot tea for everyone, which was much appreciated. Some of us ventured outside cautiously, to try to find others and make plans, but found no one. The hotel staff had departed and not turned up for work – understandably. We just sat around and waited to be rescued. I had faith in my hosts that someone would come to find me before too long. They did – or, rather, he did. A man was calling us and then he found us. It was the British High Commissioner himself, come to look for me. I was amazed but very pleased when he gathered my belongings and said to come with him at once to his house to get fed and dried.

There were two of us in my visiting team and the High Commissioner took us out to his rather battered Land Rover and, once we were inside, he said apologetically that he must go to the High Commission office before taking us home, to see that it was all right. He and his wife had been battened down for the night and were worried lest the office was flooded or destroyed, so we assented readily and looked around us at the devastation in the town. Trees covered the roads, blocking most, but already men were at work clearing them away. I have a vivid memory of a petrol station roof – a big steel one – lifted up onto its end and resting like a sail, vertically. I could not conceive the force that must have been applied to do this. Everywhere there were men on roofs, battening down torn iron to cover houses against the rain, which continued. We reached the office without too much difficulty, mostly driving through deep water. The only damage to the office was water, and there was plenty of it throughout. I know because we started to mop it up, until our host called a halt to go home for breakfast. I was thankful, being rather shaken up by the experience, and was glad to put myself in the capable and kind hands of Mrs High Commissioner, who clothed me, fed me and found me a bed.

I rested a bit but was far too excited to stay in bed long. There was work to be done and I felt I should help in the hospital, where I was sure there would be casualties. But I found this was not so: only one man had been knocked out by a falling tree. There were a few broken bones, but no deaths known then. Later, it transpired that a fishing boat had sunk in the storm, with significant loss of life and no survivors.

So what were the priorities for me? I was clearly stuck there for a few days. There was no clean water for anyone. Electricians were already working hard to establish an emergency supply. There was a British VSO water engineer in the town and I was sure that I should make efforts to get him working to restore water supplies before people started drinking polluted water, which abounded. I spent the rest of that day alongside this young man, helping and encouraging where I could. I recall following yards of pipe to find blocks and helping to test them. It took another day's hard work to get water flowing again – and then there were many leaks to repair. The impression remains of a huge and good-natured effort by the local community to overcome the problems and get on with their lives.

# Chapter 8: India 1982-84, and the UK again

In 1982, I was transferred to advising on the large India-Aid programme. I was very excited, as this was a place I had always longed to go to. It was not long before I was visiting three or more times each year and making lasting Indian friendships. I travelled throughout India to cities and rural areas. A major project that I worked on was developing primary health care services to the rural poor in some remote parts of the country such as Bihar and Orissa. I was also greatly interested by the slum improvement projects, which I write about later.

The Government of India was then rightly very concerned at the high child mortality rates in the rural areas, and they had developed a template scheme to deliver better primary health care to the rural millions. At the time, the ODA was still suspicious of Indian programmes because of the recent disaster of their enforced sterilisation programmes for rural women (part of their new family planning programme). It took a lot of persuasion and hard work to achieve a major tranche of aid money to support primary health care. I had become especially attached to the programme in Orissa, one of the poorest states of India. I worked closely with Orissa state officials and professionals and found myself applying for (and getting) a job I had helped to develop – as a health consultant, resident in the state's capital city, Bhubaneshwar, where I now went to settle.

## India opening up to me

Thus, in 1983, a further assignment overseas began, and this time in a peaceful country which I loved. Also, I felt it was not that far from Cambodia, where I wanted to return to find out what had happened. (By this time I had had contact with others of my old team. Dr Sokphan, my project deputy, had escaped with his family to France. I visited him in Paris where he had settled as a refugee with his new wife and child. He told me all the horrible things that had happened to him and his family after that day when Pol Pot took over the city of Phnom Penh. He had escaped into the forest with his girlfriend and both families and they had crossed the border into Vietnam, where they were taken to live in a refugee camp, re-educated by the communist regime, and eventually accepted to go to France, where they had relatives.)

*****

It was not an easy assignment in Orissa; the Indian Government did not much like having foreigners working in remote areas, where they could not keep a close eye; but even so, they managed to keep tabs on us pretty well. I remember once travelling in our old jeep to some remote – really remote – villages with Indian project staff. After a long hot day on the road, we sat down to an excellent Indian dinner and Dr Harish Mishra, the Project Director, and now a good friend, was called out to a telephone – there were no mobiles then. I was surprised that there was any phone at all, and was told it was a police radio speaking to him. He came back rather upset, saying he had a message for me. I could not think how anyone knew where I was! Harish afterwards said I had a message from home to say that my aunt had died that day (it had been expected). He then said, 'The police always know exactly where you are. I have to inform them whenever you go out of Bhubaneshwar.'

Once I was permanently settled in post in India, my title was 'Training Consultant to Orissa State'. My job was to:

> assist the Orissa health ministry to develop its health training facilities and centres, helping to make their training courses, including medical training, more orientated to the needs of the majority of the people living in the villages;
> assist in the establishment of a College of Nursing to raise the standard of nursing education, and increase the numbers and quality of nurses for the health service;
> establish a State Centre for Health Education to improve communication throughout the health service and with the general public;
> oversee management of the large primary health care project being funded by the British aid programme.

I was based in the project office, with full access to senior health officials, especially the Directors of Health Services and Primary Health. I attended many meetings and conferences, often championing the improvement of primary health care to the poorest, most vulnerable people throughout the huge, very poor, state. I travelled extensively many thousands of kilometres, mostly in an old jeep or in the old Land Rover assigned to me through the project. I had many adventures.

*****

My first new experience was sleeping out in Indian government rest houses. They were very basic – little more than huts, with mud floors and plaited palm walls, usually with two bedrooms, each with one large, hard, wooden bed, on which to spread mats and erect a mosquito net. My being a woman made things difficult for the men. I was graciously allocated one room and the men the other. I soon twigged that unless they slept with me, the rest of my female colleagues – mostly nurses – would be given floor space outside, so we all moved in together, Indian-style (also Cambodian-style), and we all slept together on the one bed – hot, and fighting those mosquitoes which succeeded in breaching the holes in the net. At least I got to know them all well and they forgot I was a foreigner, but not so when it came to meals.

My senior colleagues had been told they must be very careful what I was given to eat – that I would not like to eat the same as they did. The result of this instruction was woeful for me – and for them – as we travelled many extra miles for meals at government rest houses, where special cooks knew what to give me and how to cook Western food – according to them. I did gradually dispel this myth and they were amazed when I sat down with them to a true Orissa breakfast of chapatti and curry or a spread of curry and rice. I only baulked at curry omelette for breakfast. No one could believe that I just wanted the egg without the spices. At one memorable breakfast in a remote corner of the state, we stopped overnight in a small rest house, where there was an old man cooking for us. I was given various supposedly western delicacies, including chicken and duck, all mildly curried. At breakfast I had a proper omelette with white bread, fruit and coffee. On asking, I was told that the old man used to cook for visiting foreigners who came there to shoot and that the place where we were sitting had been the lookout for tigers in the past. Looking out anxiously, I was overwhelmed by a sense of history, as I thought back to my British ancestors and countrymen and women, who had served under the Raj, several hundred years before, and who had been just where I was.

I had similar emotions whenever I came across British graves in my travels in India. In Orissa, there was an old disused church in the centre of Cuttack, the former capital. There were many foreign graves, mostly of small children, but also several mothers, dying in childbirth or of cholera or malaria. Malaria was the biggest killer of Europeans. Also in the church graveyard was a memorial for a shipload of British who were coming to Orissa to work or to join families and whose ship went aground with huge loss of life from drowning. In one remote area, Phulbani District, there was a grave of three missionaries who all died from malaria, so far from home and so tragically for their families. There were most likely many I did not see, but I thought of them all often.

## Jagatsinghpur

The most important part of my job in India was to develop training for medical officers and other health-care staff (nurses and medical assistants) in primary health care delivery. In order to do this it was necessary to develop one health centre as a demonstration training centre for health workers. It was vital that it should be accredited by one of the universities/medical schools. The Indian officer who was detailed to work on this was a very committed primary health care trainer called Professor Shee. Like many Indians, he was a very hard worker, and, a bit like me, he always wanted everything to be done at once. As he was a staff member of the Cuttack Medical College, the premier medical school in Orissa, it was not too difficult to gain recognition of our training programme from that medical school. I think the authorities found the whole concept of primary health care to be rather difficult, and it tended to be thought of as second rate health care in situations where there aren't any proper doctors. Indian doctors, on the whole, were very dismissive of primary health care and they did not much like passing on skills to people they saw as other skilled workers who might possibly become a threat.

Professor Shee and I both worked hard to convince these senior personnel of the value of village-level health workers being able to provide basic health care for minor illnesses among 'the rural masses'. Professor Shee had already set up one health centre as a training ground for young doctors. So all we had to do was develop this further, to provide training for a wider range of health workers, but this meant constructing a building with several classrooms and sleeping accommodation for the students. Funding was provided by the project. The professor and I included offices for ourselves within this new training centre. It was clear that I would often have to stay overnight at the centre, therefore I asked for a small room where I could sleep. This was agreed – rather reluctantly, because there were few staff who could look after me (a helpless foreigner). In fact, I almost always stayed at a nearby government rest house. This was quite well set up, and I was comfortable there.

The training centre was about two hours by road from my house in Bhubaneshwar. It was a rather lovely drive through the countryside, especially in the early morning. I got to love seeing the ox carts, and the farmers and their families, going out to the fields to work. My driver and I used to start out very early in the morning, preferably before 6.00 am. We would arrive in time for breakfast, and to start the day's training, which usually took place at a nearby primary health centre, which entailed more driving.

We had to develop the primary health centres a lot, but that was interesting and rewarding. I found the training very challenging. Most of the young Indian doctors thought it was all an awful waste of time. Just occasionally, I came across one or more who really understood, and who I'm sure have made very good doctors now. The majority had ambitions to become specialists, especially surgeons, very quickly. In this way they could earn more money than if they remained as a primary health care centre medical officer, which was very badly paid and held in low esteem in the state.

I would love to go back to Jagatsinghpur Training Centre sometime to see if it is still there and how it developed. I have never been back, but perhaps I will. It would be interesting to see how long it lasted and what the impact was. Did I make a difference in Orissa – especially to the poorest people?

I worked almost exclusively with Orissan colleagues, but was gradually joined

172

by British consultants brought out under the project to undertake very specific tasks – for example, teaching paediatrics to medical students and teaching health education methods, or to act as senior nurse managers for the new nursing college, and nurse tutors to train local tutors. It was good to have colleagues from home to work with me. Some of them found it hard to adapt to the harsh living and working conditions, such as limited electricity, poor water and many mosquitoes.

## Land Rovers in India

Sambalpur was the capital town of Northern Orissa. It was not big or prosperous, but boasted a medical college and university, which I needed to visit as part of my job. It was a long and hot journey by road – a rough, non-tarred road over mountains and through forests – and it took 12 hours on a good day. Traffic was not much and mostly transport trucks.

One long day I was driving – or my driver was – up the road to attend a meeting. Suddenly, on a mountainside in the hot sun, there was an ominous clanking noise under my old Land Rover. It stopped. My driver was worried, as was I, and we tried everything we knew to get it going, but to no avail. We were stuck about 20 miles from our destination. One of us had to go for help. I did not fancy being left there alone; I had heard many stories of bears and even tigers in the forest. Also, I was not confident that my driver would be able to persuade someone to come out to my rescue. So I decided he should stay. I stopped the next big truck and persuaded a very surprised and reluctant driver to take me up into his cab and drop me off at a garage in Sambalpur. What a journey it was! I had not before or since driven high up in a heavily-loaded truck. It was so hot, but the view was sensational. We reached a little old garage in the centre of town and I found a sympathetic, English-speaking mechanic and described my problem. He shook his head in the Indian way and gloomily predicted big problems. After a while he agreed to go out to tow the vehicle in to his workshop. His condition was that I went with him to locate it and to pay the bills. So, back I went – in a breakdown truck. We had no problem towing the Land Rover in with the driver steering the tow. We left it in the workshop and went off very late to my meeting.

Next day it was all gloom at the garage and they told me that the shaft had broken inside something. The only remedy was a new shaft, which they did not have. They would have to send to Calcutta, some three days on the train. But I was saved by an old mechanic who appeared suddenly from the workshop interior. He said to my driver that he had worked on these Land Rovers all his life and knew them very well. He told us that he knew where there was an old Land Rover like mine buried in the mud in a nearby riverbed. He thought the shaft would be there intact, and we could dig it out quickly for the cost of the labour.

So, I was saved through the misfortune of a past British worker and I was pleased to have my vehicle on the road again in two days. I wonder if anyone else has dug up an old car to find a spare part like this?

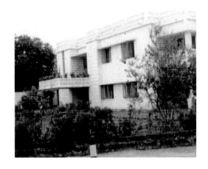

*50 Forest Park, Bhubaneshwar –*
*the ground floor was mine*

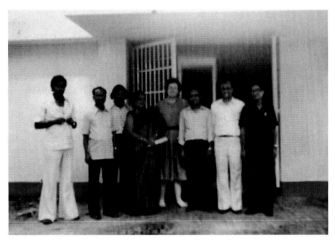

*With colleagues in Orissa, 1984*

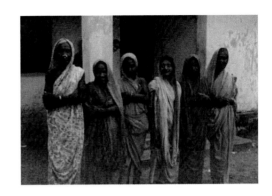

*Village traditional birth attendants*

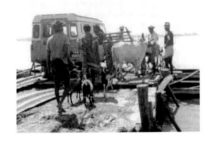

*My Land Cruiser on a local ferry crossing the Mahanadi River*

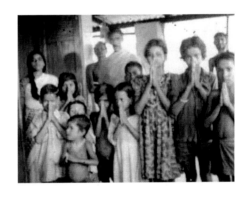

*Children at a leprosy centre, Cuttack*

I was in Orissa when Mrs Indira Gandhi was assassinated. It was devastating for most ordinary Indians, but for us in Orissa it was specially poignant as she had visited us the week before her death and I clearly remember the sight of her standing on the back of an open truck in a long procession driving proudly past my house; she had smiled and waved to me, having endeared herself to all of us over a few days. How we all mourned her loss.

For Orissa, there was a double blow. That same week, they were expecting a formal visit from HRH Princess Anne, visiting with Save the Children Fund.

175

Naturally, due to Mrs Gandhi's state funeral and all India's mourning period, that visit had to be postponed.

When the time came, a few months later, Princess Anne's visit was exciting and time-consuming. For me personally, it was a highlight: I was asked by the Palace to undertake the role of her personal physician, should she encounter any health problems. What a responsibility it was, though thankfully I was not called upon, other than socially. I had to accompany her in her train, which was an honour and a joy; she talked to the Indian officials effortlessly and was clearly interested in their work. I was able to help her a little by explaining some of the Orissan customs and I was honoured by an invitation to dine at her table one evening. She was charming and interested in all I and the Orissans were doing in our work together. When she left the local airport, she actually turned back from the gangway steps when given a sign that the plane was not quite ready, to come across the tarmac and talk to me, wishing me well in my work and saying goodbye. It was a lovely royal touch.

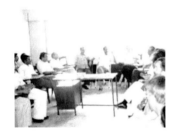

*Paediatrics course seminar*

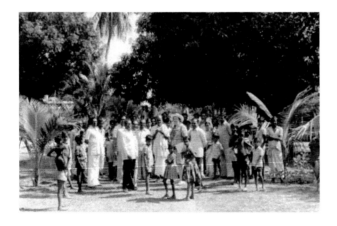

*In the community as an honoured guest*

I enjoyed living in that beautiful and still truly rural place and working at the grassroots. I could write another book about this time in my life. It all came to an abrupt end after just under two years when my father became very ill with a heart attack. I went home at once, but he died the next week. It was hard to leave my elderly mother in her grief – but a contract is a contract and I was allowed only two weeks' compassionate leave. I gave my notice for six months' time.

## Back to England – and Cambodia?

When I had worked the six months' notice, I went home to resume working with the ODA in London. Mother, who was not well, having rather given up on life after Dad died, became more and more confused. She moved to Salisbury to be near my younger brother and his family, and I went down from London each weekend to run the house for her. It was not ideal for either of us and I know she was very lonely. Alzheimer's disease was diagnosed after another year and she could not live alone any more.

Meanwhile, I had worries about not getting promoted, and had become more aware of the lack of formal public health training in my career. This awareness was mainly due to my frequent contacts with various lecturers from the UK, most of whom were staff members of either the Liverpool or London Schools of Tropical Medicine. My qualifications were not enough. I lacked expertise in epidemic and community health. Although I had plenty of field experience, which is usually much respected, I did not have the academic qualifications to progress up the ladder and became convinced that I should attempt to get my Master's degree, even though I was well over the top as far as average age goes. I was delighted when the ODA agreed to my having a paid year off and to fund my course at the London School of Hygiene and Tropical Medicine. So, after just a few months at home sorting out my life, I enrolled in September 1984 for the Master's course in community health in developing countries.

****

## Studying again: The London School of Hygiene and Tropical Medicine

I was the elder of the course by quite a few years, but no one seemed to mind that. I found it very hard to go back to lectures and examinations, although I could cope with most subjects by calling on my overseas experience (which too few of the students had), but I was very lost in the statistics course, which was the first module we took. I was given tremendous support and help by bright young men, mostly from the Indian subcontinent, who were not at all fazed by the course, nor by giving a hand to granny as she struggled to understand. I managed to pass the statistics exam at the end of the first term, and I was very relieved to pass reasonably well. If I had not, I would have had to sit it again. Then I had to tackle epidemiology, which I found interesting but quite difficult. We had a teacher who delighted in getting his students all muddled and confused. He really did try to trick us when we did mock epidemiology surveys. Again, I had to rely on course colleagues to help me out.

I studied hard, but managed to have a good time as well. I found my fellow course members very stimulating. They were mostly from developing countries such as Nigeria, Ghana and India. There were several from America and just two or three of us from the UK.

In the spring of 1985, the whole course went on a field trip to Yorkshire. The purpose of this was to carry out studies especially on water supplies and sanitation. But we also spent quite a bit of time sightseeing, and I found it very enjoyable – and we got to know each other much better. Then, right after this field trip, we had to get down to our theses. I had decided to write about something I knew well, from my time in India. I had a lot of data from all the work that I had done in Orissa, and it ended up (after several rewrites), with the title of 'Women's Health in Orissa'. (The summary of my thesis is in an Appendix to this book.) I enjoyed doing the data analysis and writing, but I knew that it had to be good in order to pass the course and gain my Master's degree. The main examinations were yet to come.

In July of that year, we sat examinations in all the modules that we had taken on the course. Again there were more statistics, but particularly epidemiology. The results would come out very quickly, and we all waited with bated breath. The system of giving results was rather cruel. We were told that any borderline cases would have to undertake a viva interview, but at the same time we were told that, if we were under consideration for a distinction, we would also have a viva interview. Thus, a list of those that were to have a viva was posted on our notice board one evening, calling for interviews next day. There was no indication as to whether the listed person was borderline for passing or being considered for distinction. They could all have been borderline, and thus in danger of failure. In fact, my name was on the board, and I was totally convinced that I was likely to fail. I remember being very upset, and only being comforted when a friendly lecturer told me that I was actually being considered for distinction. I was amazed and went home to mug up a lot of epidemiology. Now, I was determined that I was going to get a distinction. But I did not have much confidence in myself. The next day, I waited very nervously for my turn. When it came, I was not well prepared to be faced with the epidemiology lecturer who liked to tie us all up in knots (literally). He duly did just that with me. So I thought, 'That's it – no distinction for me.' But again, I was wrong and was extremely happy when I was posted next day as passing examinations with distinction, dependent on the results of my thesis. I was very proud of myself, especially because my thesis was deemed worthy of a distinction and my Master's degree was awarded 'with distinction', which I did not think too bad from the course granny!

So I returned, elated, to the ODA and was duly congratulated by my colleagues and seniors. I need not worry any more about not having the qualifications, and I felt better equipped for my public health role, as I advised Ministries of Health on developing their health systems. In fact, from this time on, when I was asked to describe what I did, I would say, 'I am a specialist in health-systems development.' I found that this terminology covered most of what I could really do and offer.

Quite soon, and for her own safety, Mother had to go into a residential home; we found a nice homely place for her back in Devon and near my brother Tim. I bought my own little house in a village nearby to see her often and I then commuted each weekend from London to Exeter and back on Monday mornings for work. Luckily, the ODA were helpful about flexitime and I was quite often allowed to do a four-day week, working from home on Fridays. My job was increasingly busy as I became more senior and my travel programme increased.

## Principal Health Advisor

By now, it was the end of 1985, and I took up my next post in the ODA. Now I was Principal Health Advisor, having been awarded my promotion as a result of doing so well on my Master's course. It was all worth it, but I had to discover what the new role meant, and found that the only difference from before was that I had to deputise for the Chief Health Advisor when he was absent from base! This turned out to be rather frequent, as he was seconded to work in Iraq for several months. I think I responded reasonably well in my new responsibility, and I enjoyed being in a position to support all ODA health advisors, wherever they were posted in the world.

Another of my duties now was to manage a large number of health research projects, which were funded by the ODA and which had to be monitored closely. I learned a huge amount about the importance of health research and its application in the field. I was particularly interested in the tropical disease research programme of WHO, with which I had a lot of contact. The ODA was a major donor to the programme, and it was my duty to lead the UK ODA delegation at the annual board meeting of the programme. I was honoured by WHO when I was asked to chair the board meeting one year. I enjoyed this and found it very stimulating and hard work.

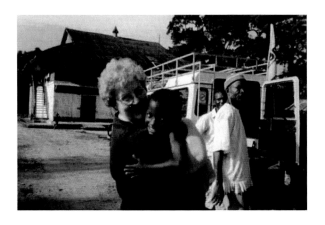

*With a young friend in Angola*

As soon as the Chief Health Advisor returned to base at the ODA, I reverted to my role as a geographical advisor and was delighted to be assigned to cover the Africa regional programme as well as the country programmes in West Africa. During the next few years I spent many months developing the ODA's health assistance programme in Nigeria and in Ghana. I made a visit to Angola, which was another post-conflict country, reminding me of the horrors of Cambodia. The ODA was being asked to fund several voluntary organisations' work programmes in Angola, and it was my job to assess their value and their appropriateness to be funded. I found I could apply my Cambodia experience quite well in this war-torn country. It was another place where many educated people, especially senior doctors and nurses, had fled to other countries, where they were welcomed. So Angola had to start to produce health service staff again. I was delighted to be able to write a very positive report in support of the proposed projects, which were duly funded, and I hope made a difference to the very vulnerable women and children in that very poor, war-torn country.

## Slum Improvement Projects

It was during this time, while other work was going on, in the years 1984 to 98, that I was very involved with ODA colleagues in advising on the health conditions and needs of some enormous slums in Indian cities. ODA had wisely decided that funding for the huge and terrible slums was well justified.

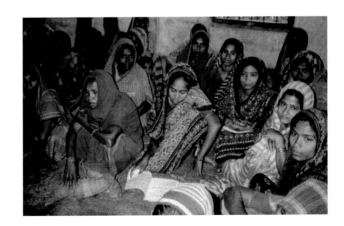

*Talking with traditional birth attendants – a women's literacy class, Jagatsinghpur 1983*

We, the health, building, engineering and social development advisers, had the job of working with Indian officials to develop projects to fund. So we visited first to see and find out; we went to Bombay, Delhi, Calcutta, Madras and other cities. I found it quite overwhelming – so much extreme poverty and suffering – so few services of any kind; no clean water, drains, schools, clinics; nothing.

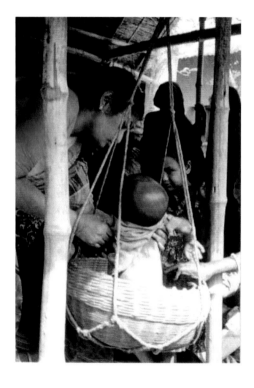

*Infant welfare –*
*India 1989*

The Government of India and of each State was trying with limited resources and manpower to tackle an immense and shameful situation. They came up with the Slum Improvement Projects (SIP). Previously they had had a policy of slum eradication or slum clearance which didn't work: the people only suffered more and went to set up a new slum elsewhere. So now the aim was to improve each slum and make it into a reasonable place to live, work and educate their children. What a huge task it was for us all. We sat down with community leaders, women and men, and tried to establish services that were appropriate and would be used.

It was slow development but over several years we saw improvements – drains and clean water, even sanitation – in schools, and in health generally. Mostly, people wanted food, houses, schools and hospitals. We were sure that priorities were clean water, clean environment and better sanitation. We had to compromise and do some of each to have a satisfied community. We did build schools and clinics, with emergency and maternity beds, but we put our major efforts into developing water supplies and providing sanitation to every house. In places where there was high child malnutrition, the government of India set up food programmes, through schools.

I went to India at least eight times just for these projects and although the work is not finished yet, as the slum cities are still there, I am convinced that we did make a difference to some slum dwellers. There were never jobs for everyone, so supporting the family was very difficult for a man. I understand why they turned to rickshaw-pulling and begging: anything to earn a few rupees for food.

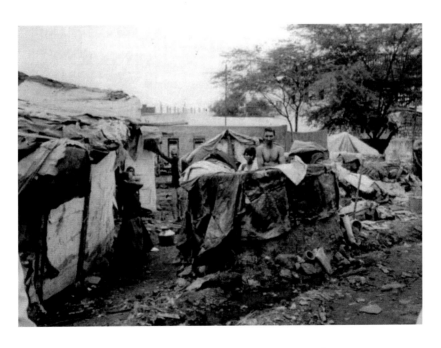

*1989–90 Hyderabad, unimproved slums*

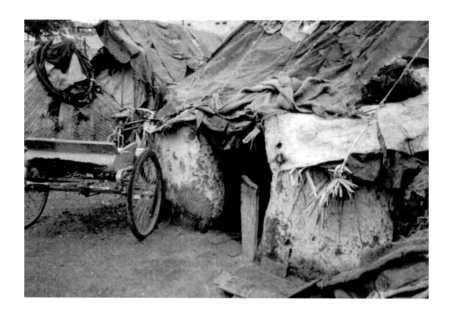

*1989–90 Hyderabad, unimproved slum dwelling*

I remained in post at the ODA for another twelve years, up to my retirement in 1998. I concentrated on health programmes in Africa and, especially, spent interesting times assisting health development in Nigeria, where services had deteriorated seriously from what had been a model for all Africa to what was now a country with excessively high mortality from infectious diseases, especially in childhood. The country was flooded with fake medicines: you could never be sure what was actually inside any pill or capsule when you bought it from a village pharmacy, market stall or peddler. HIV was just beginning and I clearly recall visiting a ward in a small district hospital and being taken by young doctors to see some patients who they could not diagnose. These were young men, all skinny and feverish, who had been labelled as tuberculosis cases – until all the tests came back negative. These doctors had never seen cases of AIDS, but they were to see many more. One of our projects involved funding hundreds of sets of AIDS diagnostic equipment all over Nigeria and then arranging training for health staff, including laboratory staff. It was tragic.

During these latter years, I visited WHO in Geneva many times, where I worked with the Emergency Unit and Tropical Disease Research

Department. I attended the World Health Assembly as part of the UK delegation, always led by our Department of Health. I was proud to know many country leaders and to introduce them to our delegates. My involvement with Tropical Disease Research was at a time when a new focus on malaria deaths worldwide was being pushed by the World Bank and UN programmes. WHO was expected to take the lead in what came to be known as the Rollback Malaria (RBM) Programme. I was so involved that I was called to work as a fulltime consultant on that programme soon after my retirement.

I was delighted at that time to visit India again to provide continuity on a few of the previous projects I had worked on. I only went back once to Orissa, but I can report that my early prediction that a five-year project was ridiculous (though too diplomatic then to put it in those words), and that a minimum of 20 years was needed to build sufficient capacity in the Orissa health services to make an impact on child mortality, appeared to have proved only too true. Twenty years after its start in 1981, the ODA was still working alongside Orissa Health Department and I still hope to revisit it one day.

*****

In the back of my mind I still thought often of Cambodia and scanned the news all the time to know what was happening. News that leaked out was all of horror and killing. Vietnam had occupied and governed the country since 1979, after defeating the Khmer Rouge. But Vietnam kept very tight control over the people and did not allow visitors or any contact with the world. Even the NGOs, Oxfam and SCF, had a difficult time trying to help, and any information came mostly from them.

# Chapter 9: Cambodia II: My first return – and Kan's story

## My first return

In 1989, the UN mounted a programme to rehabilitate Cambodia and open it up to the world. This was due to the activities of old King Sihanouk, who lived in China. The British government, along with other western countries, was allowed to send an official delegation to report on the situation and make proposals for an aid programme. Through the good offices of friends and colleagues who knew of my great interest and past involvement, my name was put forward to our Foreign Office as someone who knew Cambodia. So we set off – just four of us – on a nightmare and, for me, highly emotional, even painful, visit to my old home, that I had left in such chaos and turmoil fourteen years earlier.

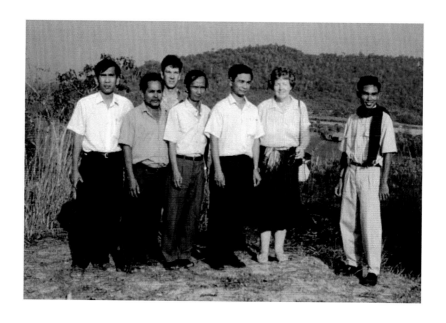

*With the planning team near Sihanoukville*

We flew to Saigon, now Ho Chi Minh City, and from there we travelled by road to the Cambodian border and thence up a badly bomb-damaged road to Phnom Penh. I could not believe I was there. I was continually searching for faces I knew – but unsuccessfully. The Cambodian government officials had all changed – most of the old regime had been violently killed after being tortured in the notorious Tuol Sleng School (Torture) Prison. Their bodies had been stacked in the killing fields – so called because of the hundreds of skulls later found buried there – on the edge of Phnom Penh.

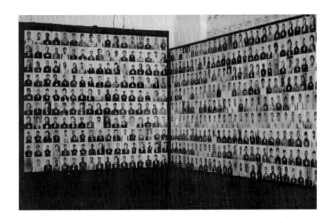

*Victims of the killing fields. These portraits were taken before Pol Pot's soldiers killed each one in Tuol Sleng Torture Prison.*

\*\*\*

I cried when we reached the city. It was totally changed. Roads were destroyed and traffic very scarce. Many beautiful old buildings had been wrecked. Only the King's Palace, Independence Monument and Central Market were untouched. Temples had been sacked. There was no mains water supply, no drainage, no electricity, and there was garbage, including old cars, everywhere. (For months I searched for my orange Mini.) We were escorted by the regime to a government guesthouse near Wat Phnom and it was almost like a prison.

I had had high hopes of being able to go out and find my friends and old team but it was impossible. We were closely guarded and not allowed out on our own. It was made clear to me that personal contacts were out of the

187

question.  However, I did find one friend among the Cambodian team escort.  I think he knew I had worked there before, and that I knew some Khmer language.  He told me he would get a message to my friends and, if they agreed, he would bring them to meet me at the guesthouse.  I was very worried lest this should cause them problems, but I knew in my heart that I should try.  Imagine my delight and emotion when, one afternoon, a knock on my door admitted Kanyaket, her two little children and her husband, Huot.  They were frightened and so thin – all of them.  We had an amazing time: getting to know the scared children, who had never seen foreigners; talking to Huot, who spoke French but no English; hearing all that had happened to Kanyaket in the long years – how near death she had been and how very poor they were now, without money or food.  Then there were all my enquiries about my other staff.  Kan did not know what had happened to most of them, but she told me of Thivan's sure death and the murder of Dr Kim Nguon, his pregnant wife and little children in the first days.  We cried a lot.  I had taken tiny presents but what they needed most was good food.  I could only give them a few dollars, which they accepted gratefully.  Then they left me – and I had no further contact until 1991, when I returned to work and live there again.

***

Kan has written her own story of her war experience, which follows soon.  My research into the outcome for my staff revealed the following, as was written for World Vision in 1989:

## World Vision Medical Team 1974

The picture was taken in 1974.  It shows most of the original Cambodian members of the World Vision Medical Team, which was led by Dr Penelope Key, then employed by World Vision Australia.  Other long-term expatriate team members included Margaret Owen, Joan Carter, Barbara Neith, Sandra Menz, Isobel Broad and Lindsay Nicholls.  The team later doubled in size to meet the huge demand for emergency care.

The team undertook a remarkable mission, providing medical and nutritional care to many thousands of Cambodian children and their mothers in the streets and refugee camps of besieged Phnom Penh in the years 1973 to 1975, right up to the evacuation of Phnom Penh by the Khmer Rouge in

April 1975. Expatriates were evacuated in the turbulent weeks before this.

Pene and Margaret finally left on 14th April 1975, taking with them twenty-five orphan children from Tuol Kork nutrition centre and the wife and children of Minh Chi Voan, the World Vision Cambodian Director.

Tragically, many of this team lost their lives, either by brutal murder or by starvation or illness during the following years. Of the twenty-nine staff in the photograph, only seven are known to be alive. We who survived this horror remember our colleagues and friends with honour and love.

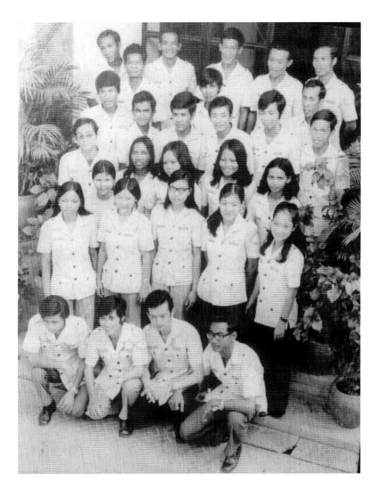

*World Vision Medical Team 1974*

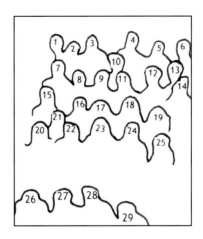

*Key to Picture*

| | | |
|---|---|---|
| 1. | Kong Chhem | alive |
| 2. | Driver ? name | died by Pol Pot 1975 |
| 3. | Long Sarun ? | died by Pol Pot 1975 |
| 4. | Prak Lam Tech | alive, working in Kratie |
| 5. | Chhim You Tech | alive, working in Calmette Hospital |
| 6. | Eng Saorin | alive, working in USA |
| 7. | Samol – driver | died by Pol Pot 1975 |
| 8. | Long Ory | died by Pol Pot 1975 |
| 9. | Thlang Samkol | alive, working in Cambodia |
| 10. | Kimsou Chantha | died by Pol Pot 1975 |
| 11. | Yap Beng Ong | died by Pol Pot 1975 |
| 12. | Dy Lamthorl | alive, working in Paris |
| 13. | ? name | died by Pol Pot 1975 |
| 14. | ? name | died by Pol Pot 1975 |
| 15. | Duong Chin Hy | died by Pol Pot 1975 |
| 16. | ? name | died by Pol Pot 1975 |
| 17. | Boun Navady | alive, living in Paris |
| 18. | Nary | died by Pol Pot 1975 |
| 19. | Kem Kanyaket | alive, living in Siem Reap |
| 20. | Sereivann | died by Pol Pot 1975 |
| 21. | ? name | died by Pol Pot 1975 |
| 22. | Lih Chung Hoa | died by Pol Pot 1975 |
| 23. | Chau Mysac | died by Pol Pot 1975 |
| 24. | Thach Thivan | killed by Pol Pot in Kpg Thom prison 1976 |
| 25. | Uy Kim Heng | died by Pol Pot 1975 |
| 26. | Dr Prum Kunthy | alive, working in USA |

| | |
|---|---|
| 27. Dr Duong Sok Phan | <u>alive, working in Paris</u> |
| 28. Dr Khvat Kim Nguon | died by Pol Pot with his wife and 3 children |
| 29. Dr Mam Bun Thol | died by Pol Pot 1975 |

*(Note: As I have been working on this manuscript, The Sunday Times has printed a comment on 06.07.08 – see <u>timesonline.co.uk/news</u>. From The Archive, they published an article by the journalist Jon Swain regarding the fall of Phnom Penh on 17th April 1975 – a date which features so much in Kan's story.*
*I have also found it interesting to read <u>Jewels of Cambodia</u> by Brenda Slogget, www.authenticmedia.co.uk ISBN 1 – 85078 – 637 – 2)*

## My Sister Kanyaket's Story

written down for her by her daughter Kannary

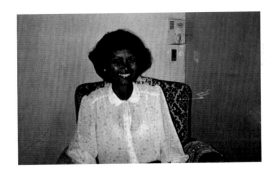

*Kanyaket*

## My First Job

In November 1973 my classmate Thach Thivan came to my house and suggested to me to go to work like her as an interpreter with a new medical team. She said it was a good salary but you have to work with the poor people. Then she arranged an interview for me the day after.

The interview by Dr Penelope Key went like this:

What is your name?

My name is Kem Kanyaket.

How old are you?

I am 25 years old.

Where did you study English?

I studied English at Beng Trabeak High School, the same school as Thach Thivan.

What are you doing now?

I am studying Literature at University and at the University of Pharmacy.

Could you come to work with my medical team like Thivan?

Yes, I would like to.

Can you come to work tomorrow?

Yes, I can.

Thach Thivan started the job one week before me. The team lacked staff, so it was not difficult for people who could speak English and needed a job. At the beginning of 1974 the team grew, with more expatriate doctors, nurses, laboratory technicians, interpreters, drivers, cleaners, and cooks. I enjoyed working during that time very much.

I am Kem Kanyaket. I finished high school at Beng Trabeak, attended first year in University of Literature and the University of Pharmacy in Phnom Penh. My father, Kem Suong, was a businessman; my mother, Penn Uttara, a housewife. My older brother Kem Atisophorn, a Polish military lieutenant; he married Ly Chev Cheng and had one son and one daughter. My brother, Kem Visetho, single, studied at the same high school as me. He won a scholarship to Australia in 1970. In 1971 he failed his exams. He wrote a letter to my parents asking, could he return home, or stay there and the family send money to sponsor his study or should he work to pay for his study? My parents decided that he should come home. In 1972, he became a trained soldier in Australia for two years. In 1974 he trained in tank attack in America for one year. He returned home in March 1975, then on 17th April 1975 all the people were evacuated by Khmer Rouge (Pol Pot) from Phnom Penh city to the rural areas of Cambodia. My brother, Kem Visetho, disappeared from the family on 25th April 1975 with Kem Atisophorn, when they went to collect food from home. Since then we've never seen them again; maybe they died?

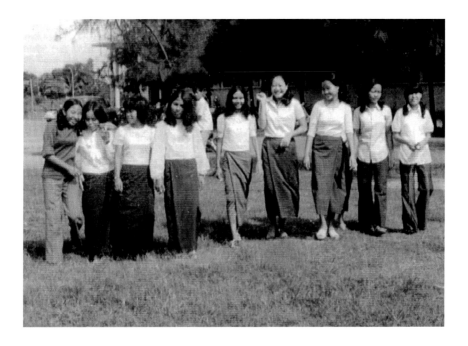

*High School students, Kan and Thivan 5th and 6th from left, 1973*

Before 1975, my sister, Kem Tolika, was a teacher, teaching in a private school. She survived; she has a husband, two daughters and one son, born after the 1979 liberation.

My sister Kem Sarany, was a student before 1975. Now she has a husband and three sons.

Kem Chino and Kem Chivo, twin brothers, died in 1977 by starvation.

Kem Youphin, my brother, survived; he has a wife but no children. He has a mental health problem, we tried to help him much but he has not improved.

Kem Chinneary, my sister, was a smart girl, but she died in 1978 of malaria and diarrhoeal disease.

Kem Kavy Ratha, my youngest sister, survived and now she has married Dr Ly Vichearavuth. She has one son, Ly Sokunthearo.

My mother died in 1978 from illness and sadness. My father now, in 2007, 89 years old, has recently taken a young wife half my age. They have one daughter 13 years old and one son 11 years old, who are my half-sister and half-brother.

## World Vision

In 1973, Dr Pene and the expatriate team were very active. We welcomed the new members employed by World Vision Australia. We worked hard at our Nutrition Centre in Toul Kork. Most children were orphaned and under 5 years old. The house in Toul Kork was on two floors. The first floor we called 'Orphanage Ward' and the second floor we called 'Emergency Ward'. I was working in the emergency ward, two days on, two days off, one month on days and one month at night. Thus I could continue my studies in pharmacy.

After one year of employment, we employees were given one month's salary as bonus. A dollar was worth a lot and the local currency was very weak.

The situation at that time in 1974 was very bad, with the noise of rocket flights everywhere in the city. Staff members of the World Vision Medical Team, which was led by Dr Pene, lived in a house on Keo Chea Street, near Sisovat High School. Every morning I came to meet my team in this house and read the schedule before going to work. World Vision's task was to help the refugees. The team undertook a remarkable mission providing medical and nutritional care to many thousands of Cambodian children and their mothers in the streets and refugee camps of besieged Phnom Penh in the years 1973 to 1975.

Because there were lots of rockets being fired into the city, students could not go to school; all the streets were quiet and there were no sellers in the markets, no TV and no radio. Khmer New Year was from 13th to 15th April. My family stayed at home. We did not celebrate because my brother's daughter aged nine months, had severe dengue fever. Dr Kim Nguon and Dr Duong Sokphan tried to save her, but sadly she died on 16th April 1975 at the Cambodian Red Cross office. (Dr Pene had transferred all the emergency children from Nutrition Tuol Kork to the Cambodian Red Cross on 10th April 1975.)

On 17th April 1975, early in the morning, my family buried the child at the corner of the house. At lunchtime, troops of black uniformed soldiers, with weapons, walked into my house and said, 'We are peaceful now – but you have to come out from your house for three days for us to organise the city.' There were black uniformed troops coming in and out of every house – some talked nicely but some were very rude. We were very scared of their voices.

## Leaving home with regret

We had three families in the large house and this is what happened to us by the end of the war in 1979:

My uncle PENN TIPO, a lawyer, died
His wife Sokha died
Daughter Penn Sithya, 26 years old, survived

195

Son Penn Panheasarik, 24 years old, died
Son Penn Visarado, 22 years old, died
Daughter Penn Thau Vanny, 19 years old, survived

My family:
Father KEM SUONG survived
Mother Penn Uttara died
Brother Kem Atisophorn died
Sister-in-law Ly Chiev Cheng survived
His son Kem Nopokun died
Myself Kem Kanyaket survived
Brother Kem Visetho died
Sister Kem Tolika survived
Sister Kem Sarany survived
Brother Kem Chino died
Brother Kem Chivo died
Brother Kem Youphin survived
Sister Kem Chinneary died
Sister Kem Kavy Ratha survived
Auntie Penn Ponnakry died
Cousin Ros Boneau died
Cousin Ros Moly died

My uncle KUOCH BUN RITH died
Auntie Penn Vuthy Samphea died
Son Kuoch Bun Cheang died
Son Kuoch Bun An died
Daughter Kuoch Ammara died

It was 17th April 1975, time to pack up and leave. All of us understood that we were leaving home only for three days, and then we would return home. So we took only necessary things like rice, food, money and our personal jewellery – gold and precious stones like rubies, emeralds and diamonds that were mined in Cambodia. But some jewellery of relatives who wanted us to keep it for them, we could not take with us.

Khmer Rouge propaganda had all been about liberation and peace. I packed only two or three dresses that I liked; I put everything in order carefully. I did not take my make-up with me. I prepared my bed, my books, my photographs very well. I loved my room very much.

All of us came, walking out from the house; we left our car at home. We carried rice – about 10 kilograms; dry fish – 2 kilograms; noodles – two boxes; pots and a frying pan for cooking. We saw some people brought their car and lots of goods, which looked very strange to us. Why didn't they leave them in their house? Because in three days the Khmer Rouge would allow us to return home.

From my home to Monivong Bridge was two kilometres. The Khmer Rouge asked us to go far down from the city before dark. My uncle's family followed my family, but auntie's family went separately to her husband's village in far off Battambang Province.

After three days there was no news about returning home. The black uniformed troops said 'Now King Sihanouk has returned to Cambodia, we need all the military Generals and Lieutenants to return to the city for re-organising the country.' My two brothers, in patriotism, left the family behind, then walked with Khmer Rouge troops. We were waiting for them for five days without news at the Niroute Pagoda. (We learned later that many who went back were straightaway executed.) Then I met with Dr Duong Sokphan and his family at Niroute Pagoda. Dr Sokphan told me not to stay longer, and that I should encourage my family to go to Vietnam with his family. We refused, because we could not speak Vietnamese like his family. The Khmer Rouge chased us away from that place and said, 'You should go to your own village.' Our group together had twenty-one members, so then we had to make our own shelter at Prek Ang Village route number 1. There was rain, no hygiene, no good water to drink, people got cholera. We saw death everywhere and it was smelly. We had registered in the Khmer Rouge records that we would go to Kompong

Cham, my father's home town. My mother did not like to go, because her two sons had not returned yet. She was crying every day for fear of losing them. We were missing our home so much; our hearts were breaking and full of regrets.

## Motorboat to Kompong Cham Province

Bye, bye, Phnom Penh! Tears non-stop. We were very shocked and we cried a lot. In my group there were two old men, three old women, nine girls, six boys and one little boy, missing my two brothers, so the total was twenty-one members.

The fast boat reached the bank called 'Chihee' and we had a reception from Khmer Rouge soldiers. They said, 'Angka takes care of you to liberate you from the reactionary conservatism, so you must be grateful to Angka.' We had not had enough food to eat for one month; this time we ate too much. Then they put us in an ox-cart to find my father's parents.

*\*\**

We rested with the relatives for one week, then Angka separated us into small huts; they called us 'the refugees of 17th April' or 'a new people after liberation'.

During the evacuation period, Khmer society seemed to be in disarray. People tried to find their way out of the city or chose to go to their home town. Everywhere things seemed to be very quiet. The Khmer Rouge threatened that if anyone was hiding the enemy (generally foreigners, soldiers of the old army, or government people), the whole family would be executed. All of us were very nervous.

The Khmer Rouge did not allow us to walk, or to contact people, and at night we were told, 'Do not talk, Angka will patrol.' I was sent out to work with a single group, male and female separated. Middle-aged male with male, female with female, old lady to take care of babies, grandpas to make baskets. The amount of food we received depended on how many family members there were and how much work each of them could perform. There was never enough food.

We lived near a flood area. My relatives told us, 'Water will come in November and last for about forty or fifty days.' During that time we needed to stock firewood and reserve food to eat. My uncle lived with nine family members in his hut. My family lived with twelve members in our hut.

We were working hard at daytime, and at night we could not talk to each other. Every day and night we prayed and thought only about food, because our stomachs were starving. After the flood finished we, the 17th April group, were sent out to different regional places.

## Moving to Kampong Thom Province, Stuong District

Early in 1976, the restrictions of the Khmer Rouge army got worse and worse. Boys and girls must cut their hair short; they had no colourful clothes, only black. We had to dye our clothes black. We did not have many clothes to change. When something was torn, we cut from one garment to sew a patch on the other. If you worked hard, Angka provided a shirt, skirt, scarf, shoes, trousers and cotton bag.

We worked from five o'clock in the morning until dark. We got to rest for only ten minutes twice a day. The people who smoked had the chance to smoke just one cigarette until finished. There were many men and women who pretended to smoke.

After three months in Stuong, Khmer Rouge army caught my uncle (he was a lawyer) and tied him up to be killed. They said, 'If you are former soldiers, former police officers, CIA agents or KGB members, you are the enemy of the revolution.'

Three days later at night the army caught my cousin Ros Boneau because Angka was not satisfied with him and did not like him, so he had to be killed. His sister Ros Moly was sad and cried all the time. The army sent her to a district clinic in the temple. After two months she wasn't better so they sent her to the district hospital. She did not eat; she looked very ugly, like a skeleton, with deep eyes, deep chin and low voice. We visited her, and tears came from her eyes. She said, 'I will not see you for ever – I will die soon.' Then one night she drank all the medicines that the nurse gave her, to poison herself. She died that night. We collected her body and buried her in the pagoda. My auntie became ill after her husband was caught. She had diabetes, but there was no treatment and so she became very weak and died. We buried her in that pagoda too.

Our family was working very hard, but we were blamed every time. We were trained how to spread rice seeds in the fields or plant rice on the hard soil. After sowing, we pulled up the young plants to plant in the field. We were forced to work non-stop without enough food; all day and night under the sun and in the rain. We walked without shoes everywhere, on dirty mud or rock or forest. That time my feet were swollen. Tolika and Sarany had the same problem as me, Chino was wounded by leeches eating his leg. It was bleeding and smelly and looked like an ulcer. The army looked down on him very much. We were all in the nursing house treating him. One morning Chino woke up and walked down to the garden. When he came back, he carried a fat death lizard in his hand. He was very happy; he said, 'It is for lunch today.' Suddenly, while he climbed the stairs, he fell down, so we helped him to his mat to lie down on the pillow. He started to talk, saying, 'Hopeless! My life will end today.' The situation was terribly sad; he begged the Khmer Rouge chief, 'Could you please give me one cup of milk and one bowl of rice, please?' That woman did not like to provide it; she said it was too late; his pulse was weak, he closed his eyes. He took half a day to pass away. We buried his body in the same pagoda. After we had nursing treatment, we got better, so we went back to work again in the field.

One month later, Angka Top appointed me to the battle field in Kampong Thom. The rice fields were full of mines. I worked from 5.00 am until midnight. They asked me to make a channel for the rice fields – about a thousand hectares. It was very dangerous when they dug up the mines. Some died and some were wounded. I was lucky because I carried soil to make channels. My group was clever; we were originally from Phnom Penh; we were careful; when we suspected anything, we reported to the army and we were changed to another place. Many times I was lying down in the field to escape. I prayed to God quite often. We finished the channel, and Angka instructed us to go back home for the harvest season. Therefore I met my family again. My dad and mom were skinny, and my four sisters busy at the harvest far from home. Only my sister-in-law stayed with my parents. Her son Kem Nopokun died from a big stomach full of worms. He had fever, and vomited worms, but some worms got into his lungs. Kem Chivo was dying of starvation. He ended his life sitting under a tree, but no one thought he was dying.

Angka appointed me again to meet the regional workers in 1978. My mom didn't like me to go; she was afraid that I would not be with her when she died. But it was not easy to refuse Angka's instructions as Angka would probably kill me.

My main camp was in the forest, but it was only half-ready. Angka said to stop there and I had to arrange to cut trees for my own shelter in the dark. In the morning, when the sun shone, I packed and folded a mat, when suddenly I saw a snake move away from under my mat. So I knew that last night I slept on the snake – I was so scared. Angka collected all the people, especially the 17th April from Phnom Penh, living in different districts of Kampong Thom Province, to dig a main dam at Kompong Thmor District, they called it '1st Makara Dam'. My two cousins, Penn Panheasarik and Penn Visarado, and the girl named Somethy were with me. Probably about 2,000 or 3,000 people were sent to build the channel and dams.

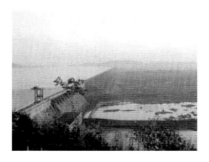

*Hirakud Dam*

Angka separated the female group five hundred meters away from the male camp. Fortunately, I met Thach Thivan there. She had changed her name to 'Mith Na', which means 'Comrade Na'. We met each other and cried. Thivan asked the group chief if she could move from her place and sleep with me, so then we got together.


## Thach Thivan

On 17th April 1975, Thivan and Dr Mam Bun Thol (our team doctor) went to work as usual at the International Red Cross house. She said the road was quiet, but the Khmer Rouge army with black uniforms occupied everywhere. Then Dr Mam Bun Thol brought her back to her home and he went. It was late for her, and her parents had left her behind. Hopeless, she did not have keys to get into the house, nothing to change or to eat. She joined a group of people, begged for food and clothes. Then she met Dr Mam Bun Thol's cousin; she was alone too. Both of them made friends and lived together until I came. She allowed Thivan to come with me, because I was more important than her. In the daytime we could not communicate; we had to concentrate on their rule. At night, before we slept, Thivan told me about her love story with Dr Mam Bun Thol... In the days when we were working for World Vision, he fell in love with Thivan; he bought some jewellery for her such as a ring, earrings, necklace with a very beautiful diamond pendant and bracelet. Now she was keeping this jewellery in a small pocket of her underwear shirt. While she worked, an army girl remarked that Thivan may be a member of 'KGB' or 'CIA' agents. I always told her to be careful, but she did not listen to me. I was very scared when she spoke English to me. She always went out to search for her family or other friends in the different camps. She called me to go with her too, but I went only once, then I stopped. About three months later, Angka told Thivan and other girls that Angka wanted them to go back to the village next day.

Thivan complained to Angka: 'Why not send Kan to go to her village too, because Kan is getting older now?' Angka replied, 'Comrade Kan – stay, Comrade Na – go!' That night Thivan could not sleep, but we could not talk to each other, because we heard someone guarding us. Early next morning, Thivan packed up her stuff and said bye, bye, to the group. I and the other comrades in the group went out to dig soil to make the dam as usual. Darkness came and Angka returned with those who went with Thivan. The army chief gave me a letter from Thivan. She said, 'Comrade Na is in Kompong Thom now, and tomorrow a truck will drive her home.' I put the letter in my pocket. I did not show my emotion of missing Thivan to them. I was crying in my heart, my soul not with me at that time. I prayed to God to bless Thivan. One day later, my friend Somethy, who came from the same village as me, told me that they found Thivan's bag, shoes, and clothes under the bed of a top army officer (she was in charge of the 300 girls). So everybody said the three comrades from yesterday were already killed. Thivan wrote to me in a red pen that she had borrowed from the army there. She said I was her best friend, she could not forget me

203

ever and was thankful for everything. She wished me good luck, good health. After I finished reading, I dug it into the ground, and pretended not to cry.

***

After Thivan left, Somethy tried to get close to me. All the time, Angka asked about the background of individuals. We always reported to each other about the questions and replies. So we had in mind to answer what we should lie or tell the truth to Angka. I told my background to Angka, and here I have written the truth in ordinary print, but the made-up story is in italics: *I was born from a poor family. Father was a worker;* mother was housewife; I had five brothers and five sisters. I was the second daughter. *I was married since 1974; my husband was a person that built houses in the countryside;* I was a tailor. I had no children. *My husband was occupied in the war in 1975 in Kompong Som. I didn't know where he was. I was 29 years old. I had been ill; I had pain and discharge from my uterus and I had stomach ache.*

Although I was very tired from the hard work, I still carried on doing my crochet or knitting for Angka. I had a favourite T-shirt bought by my brother from Australia. It was wool with stripes of colour: yellow, green and black. I cut off the collar and pulled out the wool thread in different colours. Then I made a crochet covering for a torch or radio. It looked very beautiful. So that was very attractive to Angka. They asked me to make more for them and they gave dried meat or dried fish for me to eat. I told them I can do a sock, shirt, pants or gloves for a baby from newborn until one year old. So sometimes they kept me in a place to finish what they asked me to do.

One day Angka gave all of us a new black uniform, but the size was big and long, so I said I could make it nice for them to wear. I made one for them and it was so good, so the others gave their shirts to me to make good for them too. Each day I carried about ten shirts on my head down to the village to get to the sewing machine. It was lucky for me and the army fed me well that week. I went downtown feeling so sad. In the village, there were houses, but no people living in them. There were roads, but no traffic or no people walking. There were schools, but no students or teachers. There were pagodas, but no monks. There was money, but it was useless. Every day Angka forced us to work as animals or machines. We never had soap, medicines, or light. We were living in the dark as in a jail. Angka hated the intelligent; Angka needed only illiterate people. So life was very short for us, especially the men could not survive. I was at so many camps, and again they moved me – to the hospital in Kompong Thom Province. My friend Somethy had the same illness as me and five girls got malaria. At first, all of us were in the general medical ward. Nurses called me and Somethy to see an army doctor who had had training by the Chinese.

I was lying on an operation bed. Around me were two nurses and one doctor (I guessed). The doctor put his finger on my middle and asked me, 'Did you feel pain in your feet or not?' I said yes. He read in his theory book and said to his friends, 'Give me a plastic thread with needle.' Then he put the sewing needle on the mark in my belly and cut. He kept the 2 cm thread in my skin. After that, he marked points on both my legs, then put the sewing needle in again and left 2 cm in each. I let them do it; I didn't care; I got fever so they gave me a traditional pill for treatment and gave me one injection from a drink bottle – it was pink, and I heard that it was vitamin B12 made by Angka. I was scared, because the injection was very dangerous if put in the wrong place. God blessed me! I was fine. [Pene says that Kan told her this story many times, and perhaps the treatment was a form of acupuncture.]

Two days later, Angka sent me and Somethy to the maternity ward. There were lots of senior army wives waiting to deliver their babies. We were lucky again, because Somethy helped a mother express her breast to get milk for the baby, and she gave a lot of food to us. A nurse was called for consultation about my uterus and gave me a traditional pill. We stayed in that ward only three days and they sent us to a general ward again. We went out very often around the hospital and we heard a horse-rider dragging the dead from Kampong Thom High School to be buried in the pagoda. Angka used the school as a prison. Sometimes there were only a few dead and the horse ran very fast; sometimes there were many dead and the horse ran very slowly. Imagine all those who had been killed by Angka, the Khmer Rouge.

***

We were in the hospital about a month. Then Angka brought us back to camp. This time we were moved to work in the rice fields in Kampong Thom Province. Daily we looked after the dry fields, dug channels to water the rice field. If the field was too full of water, we emptied the water away. At night-time we killed rats from the rice field. Angka asked each person to kill five to ten rats before going to bed. Poor me! I never killed even one. When I saw rat, I ran away and cried. Now at harvest time, we were in the rice fields. They were forcing us to harvest rice urgently to send to China, so we did not expect to eat our produce. Angka said to me, 'You are older than these girls. You must go back to work in the village with the middle women.'

Angka planned to break off fighting next month – I thought maybe in September 1978, before the festival of Pyom Ben. Angka released the old people to go back home. I was allowed to go back too. In the truck there were twenty women, including me. I was very silent and sad. I prayed to God to bless me, to arrive home and not be killed.

***

Fortunately, the driver stopped at Stuong District (my home district) and dropped me. He reported to Angka at Stuong that I had successfully completed hard work in Kampong Thom. The district chief welcomed me, cooked a delicious meal for me to eat. I was still anxious; why did they not say I can go to meet my family? I slept there for one night, until 10.00 am, and then they let me go. Oh my God, I breathed, I felt better...

I did not walk, I ran and ran, I missed everybody in my family. The first person that I met was my poor father. Dad was very thin. He did not wear a shirt, he had a scarf around his neck, his dirty short pants were full of holes, no shoes, he had shaved all his hair. I called my Dad from my throat and cried. He held me and cried too, 'Daughter Kan, you have long life, God bless you for coming.' We went up the steps to climb into the house. He told me Mom had died since I left her two months ago. Sister Chinneary died a month later. She had diarrhoea and starvation. Youphin in the village carried cow dung and dead leaves to make fertiliser. Tolika was sent to dig a line in the rice field with the middle women. Sarany, Pen Sithya, Pen Vanny were with the teenager group planting rice. Ratha was sick and staying in the nursing home in the pagoda. So my dream came true! While I was in Kampong Thom Hospital, I had dreamed I was back home; I did not find my Mom – she had disappeared. I searched for my sisters and I heard that Chinneary had died, but Ratha was alive. Actually, Ratha was so skinny; I never thought she could survive.

I was already sad when I returned home. I decided I would shave my hair off in gratitude for my parents. I did not like myself then. I wanted to be as ugly as possible. In the morning, I asked my Dad to shave my hair. My Dad took a sharp knife and put it on the middle of my head and only shaved one line, then was trembling. He called the neighbour to finish it.

***

I had rest for one day, then Angka sent me again to join the group of my sister Kem Tolika. Auntie Penn Ponnakry had handed over the jewellery to Tolika. There were a set of rubies, sapphires and emeralds, a belt made of gold and a Buddha also made of gold. It was together about one kilogram. Tolika kept it in her bag, mixed with some spare clothes and the mosquito net. She used the bag as a pillow. Before I arrived, she slept in the same mosquito net with a lady from 17th April. The lady was about 35 years old, and Angka had killed her husband because he was Chinese-Khmer. Her son, a teenage boy, was far away from her. Tolika had shown her the jewellery once. While I was there, Tolika told her friend that she wanted to separate from her. That lady agreed and made her own mat with mosquito net. The second day after we returned from work, we brought a lot of snails and crabs from the rice fields for our food. Tolika said, 'Wait, sister Kan, I would like to get a pin and small silver fork from my bag to take the soft body from the shell.' After a while Tolika came to me and asked if I had seen her small jewellery bag. I said, 'No, what's happened?' Tolika's face looked terrible and full of sorrow. We could not eat the food, we talked to each other to find the solution. Angka heard someone stole our jewellery. So Angka advised us, 'Comrade, not to worry, Angka will find it for you, but it will not belong to you anymore. Angka will keep it.' Angka wanted everybody equal. That afternoon, the Khmer Rouge informed us we must all be out in the field, no one to stay in the camp. In the field we were working, suddenly the suspected lady said, 'I have a headache – I need to go back.' That one army person told Tolika and me, 'Tonight, if Angka calls anyone, the other should be quiet.' That night we did not sleep well. It was midnight, and two soldiers came to awake that suspected lady and took her outside, I supposed, because we could hear the stick hitting her – about six or seven metres away. At 4.00 am the soldiers brought her back with chains on her ankles and wrists. Poor lady, she did not say one word and did not look at us. At 6.00 am we went out to work and at lunchtime we came back. We received our rice porridge as usual, then we went to rest in the hut. The lady was lying down; her wrists had been locked by the chain to the bamboo floor and her ankles were locked too. Angka came in with the bowl of rice porridge; they unlocked the wrists for her to sit and eat. She finished one bowl and Angka locked her wrists again. In the afternoon, we went to work, and when we returned, she was there. When it was dark, we went to sleep; about midnight the soldiers came and took her away and she disappeared from that time.

Three days later our group were sent in a new direction. This time I was in an agriculture group. Angka gave ten hectares of land to plant vegetables. The garden was near the river. Every morning I had to carry water buckets on my shoulder 100 times from 5.00 am until 11.00 am. In the afternoon we dug in the ground – what was supposed to be a grave for us, I thought.

At the end of December 1978, a strange event happened. We had an appeal from a lady called 'Touch'. She said, 'I am a Lotus fairy. All of you will be back in Phnom Penh next week. If you want to call me again, bring the lotus on the day of the full moon, and I will talk with you.' We were very excited after we heard that, because we longed to return to our home. The second time she appeared, she had fever, she could not go to work but rested in the hut upstairs. We were eating lunch downstairs, below where her bed was. The spirit came on her again; she was jumping on the bed, and dust got in our food. We rushed to watch her. She told us again, 'You are all lucky; you will go to see the Royal Palace quite soon.' The soldier came to ask what was happening to Comrade Touch. If she had energy, let her have a competition of digging one square metre of soil with him. Touch came out with her hoe; the soldier measured the area for them both. Touch was very strong; she dug so fast and finished it before the soldier, then she went to bed quietly. That was from the spirit, I believed, because Touch got fever and was very weak, so she could not eat and work.

Now a word that Touch told us came true. One day later we saw the helicopter flying around our village many times. Angka soldiers called for a meeting and rushed out from their families to hide in the forest or mountain. This was the first time we really knew we were to be liberated.

***

Tolika and I packed our stuff and ran to see our family. I went to see Sarany and Ratha, to hold their hands, and said we must go back to Phnom Penh. The ancient people were allowed to kill pigs, cows, chickens and distribute food to us. They divided rice from the stock until it was finished. My family prepared food to go. My Dad asked me to call Penn Sithya and Penn Vanny to join the journey with us, but they had gone with the other people.

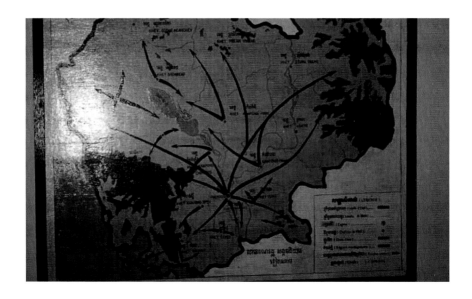

*Map showing forced migration patterns 1975-77*

### Freedom to choose

My Dad made a trailer to carry the food and rice. We chose to go back to Phnom Penh. We were now seven members: Dad, Kan, Cheng, Tolika, Sarany, Youphin and Ratha. We walked from Stuong to

Kampong Thom Province. Some people walked from Stuong to Siem Reap Province, then escaped to Thailand.

We could walk only five kilometres each day. We could not walk on the road when it was so hot because we did not have shoes. We travelled at night-time and early in the morning. We needed to cook twice a day. We travelled with many people, in terrible conditions, with many sick, having lost their family in an orphanage, now suffering a painful life. We thought there was nobody else like Pol Pot in the world. Pol Pot's policy was to kill all the people.

Living conditions started from zero; they were now most basic:
- no electricity: we used lamps with fish oil, and firewood, living in the dark;
- no spoons to eat with: we used palm leaves or a hand. Sometimes when we had one bowl of soup in the middle, we used to pass the soup round to eat one by one;
- no plates: we used coconut shells, or a gourd, or whatever we could find;
- no pen and no paper to write, so we wrote everything by hoe and long knife in the ground;
- the human being was a machine;
- no soap: we used ashes to wash hands; we used the bark of kapok, burnt then mixed with water, to make something like shampoo.
- males and females had head- and body-lice;
- skinny bodies, bloated stomachs, hollow eyes, pale swollen faces...

All the time I was in the Pol Pot region, three years, eight months and twenty days (17th April 1975 until 7th January 1979), I never had my menstrual period. As soon as we were returning, it started again, maybe because I was happy and hopeful. I did not have any sanitary napkin to change.

For the seven of us, we cooked rice in ten little tins and a very big pot of soup vegetables. Luckily, it was harvest-time and we got rice from

primary school there. She got paid in rice and shared it with the family (Dad and me).

After a week, Youphin and Ratha visited us. They informed us that they had got accommodation and we must go to stay with them there. My Dad said he could not leave Sarany alone, so he would stay there with her and I, Kan, could go and look after the sisters.

\*\*\*

Oh, Phnom Penh, I missed you so much! My dream came true; I love Phnom Penh deeply in my heart.

A pile of dead cars of different models, masses of rubbish, the smell of faeces and dead animals and bodies. There were empty houses, but some houses Khmer Rouge had used as a warehouse. In the compound around Central Market, Pol Pot had planted coconut trees, and it was fertilised by the bodies of dead soldiers. Pol Pot had killed the generals of the army and the police and buried them there. Inside Central Market, there were lots of fancy armchairs, sofas, tables of all kind of woods – they were all collected in the hall. The goods that were stored there had disappeared from somewhere before. I visited Orusei Market and I saw lots of sewing machines of all kinds – maybe a thousand. I saw many pairs of different shoes, a pile of utensils... I had been to my own house near District 6, Praw You Vong Pagoda. It remained as before, the gate was unlocked, all the doors and windows were closed, but unlocked. The furniture was gone. On the ground floor was a stack of about fifty televisions. I could not find any photographs of my family. I was afraid to stay there, although four families of us lived there before. In front was one road and behind the house another road. It was a big plot of land.

My grandfather, Khem Penn, was the formal secretary for King Norodom Sihanouk. He retired in 1959 and Grandpa died in 1962. On the day of his funeral, there were forty police and army representatives to pay respect to him. Grandpa worked in the Royal Palace.

My Aunt Penn Ponnakry was single; she worked in Sothearos School, and beside that she worked for Princess Samdech Preah Reach Kanitha Raksmey Sophorn. So with these roots, my house was like a hotel. My parents had ten children on one floor, with my Aunt Penn Ponnakry. Uncle Penn Tipo, his wife and six children (Sithya's family) were on another floor, and Aunt Penn Vuthy Samphea, her husband and three children on another.

When I returned to see my own house, I was very sad. I thought I should come back to stay, but I had to leave it a while, because it was quiet, with only a Vietnamese soldier around to chase the Khmer Rouge away.

In June 1979, I stayed in a flat at the Old Market or Psar Chas with my sister Tolika. People needed food urgently, so all of us had to register with the Community Group. My sister and I got work at the Ministry of Business to clean roads and guard the warehouses. The country was full of rubbish; it was dirty and some places smelt of sewage. Our duty was to stop people from taking goods that had been kept from the occupying Khmer Rouge soldiers.

Vietnamese soldiers were still around to help Cambodians re-establish the country. We worked with a solidarity community group and collected food every day from the main community kitchen. This time we were not starving as we had been under the Khmer Rouge regime. We had plenty of food for the whole family and old people did not have to work. The Cambodian Republic Government fed us very well. We did not get any salary. We started from zero, with nothing in our hands at all.

My family didn't like to return to our own home in Phnom Penh, near the Monument of Independence, District 6, because at that time it was not secure; especially there was no water or electricity. My father wanted to live in his own home very much. However, we decided to leave our home and live with the solidarity group.

In September 1979, I was appointed to the Faculty of Medicine. There were about sixty former students who returned to study, more women than men. The Faculty of Medicine was supervised by the Ministry of Health (MOH). Every day the MOH sent two trucks to collect us students to clear drugs from the warehouse along Kampuchea Krom Street and transport them and put them in order at the Central Pharmaceutics Control (CPC) or the Laboratory. We did that job for nearly three months.

In November 1979, all students started to learn about politics in the Faculty of Medicine, then a month later we did Technical Studies. I could not attend the classes for long, because the MOH needed me to work. In my CV, I wrote that I had finished high school at Khmer English School and had studied the first year at the Faculty of Pharmacy and the Faculty of Literature, and also I had had a job with World Vision, from 1973 to 1975, where my boss was Dr Penelope Key. As a result, the MOH appointed me to work in the Exterior Relations Office. I was translator and interpreter for the English Department. No salary was paid; all staff received meals instead. We did not have enough clothes to wear. If we did not have it yet, the Government provided accommodation.

All people had to register in the solidarity community group. In that period all people had to work together in a group and get food from the solidarity group. It was similar to a socialist/communist country. The Government distributed land or houses to all people, counting how many members in a family. It was supposed to be 150 square metres per person and if you had more area than that, you would have to pay tax in the future.

In 1980 the Government published currency notes. So then we had to manage our living conditions by ourselves. There were some markets selling fish, chicken, vegetables and fruits, but not many sellers. At that time, payment was higher for the workers than for educated people.

One time I remember a lady who was working in the MOH told me someone was falling in love with me and he asked her to inform me about him. I refused; I told him to look for a young girl, because I thought I was too old to get married and it was too late to have a baby. That man did not change his mind. After many months, I reported to my father, who then agreed to accept him as a son-in-law. Then on 24th October, 1980 I was married to Mr Kim Huot.

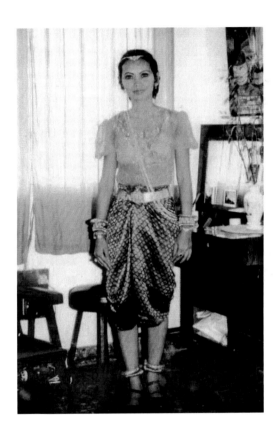

*Kan on her wedding day, 1980*

Mr Huot was a teacher. He taught mathematics in Tuol Tom Pong High School. In 1972 he had one son and in 1974 he had one daughter. In 1975, the Khmer Rouge separated him from his loving family and sent him to Kompot Province. His wife and the two children were sent to work in the fields in Battambang Province. Unfortunately, they could not survive because they missed Mr Huot too much. Mr Huot had very bad experiences in the Khmer Rouge regime; he would have died if there was no revolution on January 7th, 1979.

Three months after our wedding, we moved from a house at the Old Market to live in a flat near the MOH. This accommodation was given by the MOH for staff to live and work close by. On August 2nd, 1981, I had a son, Huot gave him his name: Huot John Kanya. He was a healthy baby, delivered in December 2nd Maternity Hospital. Huot was away for a week in Russia, working at a peace conference, and he left me alone with the baby. Srun, Huot's sister, came to help me for one month then she went home. Time flew and I had to go back to work. I dropped my son at the MOH Day Care Centre at 7.00 am and picked him up at 11.00 am; in the afternoon I dropped him at 2.00 pm and picked him up at 5.00 pm. I worked eight hours a day.

It was our family responsibility to feed three cousins of Huot who lived with us; we found a school for them. We never had enough food to eat; we were both very skinny. One of my sisters, Ratha's, husband left her eight months after she had a baby, so I had to help her and requested a job with the MOH for her, and then she came to stay with us too. In 1983 I had a baby daughter, Huot Kannary, so my family increased to nine members. The living conditions were very poor, but in 1984 two of Huot's cousins could not pass their exam, so they returned to their home. We were reduced by two, but we got one more niece. That was Chhun's sister; she wanted to come to study at school in Phnom Penh. We lived in a small flat; in one corner the four of us lived; in another corner was Ratha and her son Ro; our niece Chanry had one small bed and Chhun one small bed. Every day our meal was only a big pot of vegetable soup with some rice.

In 1985, I was quite ill; the MOH (Ministry of Health) allowed me to go for treatment in Hungary for six months. After that, I felt much better. My living conditions were very bad. I borrowed money from the neighbours every month. I sold most furniture that I had collected; I sold everything – such as plates, spoons, electric wire, milk powder provided for the baby, clothes. Sometimes I sewed school clothes to sell in the market; sometimes I had jewellery from friends to sell; then I had a commission from it. Earning money was very difficult.

Ro and John were similar ages, but Ro was six months older. When John, Ro and Kannary went to primary school, I felt released from payment to the kindergarten. Poor hungry kids – if they wanted to eat something, I always told them, 'I do not have money for you, but if you are hungry, you should help me to earn money; for example, you could sell empty bottles or empty cans to the collection men.' We had only rice soup with vegetables, a few eggs and chicken-blood or fish-paste with cucumber, morning glory, ginger, aubergines, and baby corn. We had a big responsibility to feed so many people: sister, brother, nephew, niece and our children. I was ill all the time.

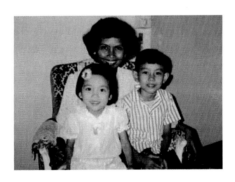

*Kan, John and Kannary 1989*

In 1989 I received a message from Dr Penelope Key via a guide from the Ministry of Foreign Affairs to make an appointment for me to meet her in the government hotel near Wat Phnom. I was so excited to meet her that time. I was not scared as before; I thought if I was killed, 'let it be'.

I asked permission from the security guards and showed her name card, so the police security guard went to call Dr Key. She came down to meet me and we were holding each other very tight and crying very loudly for five minutes, then we asked for permission to go upstairs to talk in her room. Dr Pene Key asked me to come again with the two kids every day for her three days' mission. We were so delighted and happy. She contributed some money for my family. She gave toys and clothes for John and Kannary. Dr Pene told us that she would come again soon. She wanted to work in Cambodia very much.

(end of part one of Kan's story)

***

## Pene's story continues

To return to my trip to Cambodia in 1989. In my report, I made a number of recommendations for the British Aid effort in Cambodia. This I had been asked to do as part of my Terms of Reference. It had become all too apparent that the overwhelming need was for human resource development; that is, replacement of many skilled people who had been killed or lost. There were now very few skilled doctors, surgeons, obstetricians, and paediatricians. The child mortality was huge though uncounted. The health services were in disarray and diseases such as malaria, tuberculosis, diarrhoea and even leprosy were common killers at every age. So my broad recommendations were to support the health sector, education sector and training of leaders, including English language training. We also recommended opening a VSO programme immediately, to contribute to the language situation as well as in technical training and assistance to the further development of the limb-fitting workshops and mine-clearing programme.

## Continuing and developing contact with Cambodia

When I returned to UK and the ODA after this trip, I could not get Cambodia out of my mind and my dearest wish was to go back and spend time helping there. Then it was that I began to feel seriously guilty about my life and survival. This guilt persists to this day. I knew then that I must give something back to my dear friends to make some reparation for what they had gone through.

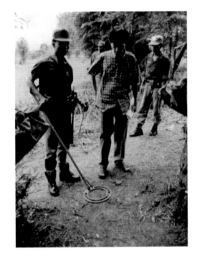

*Clearing mines*

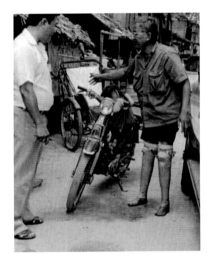

*Mobility for an ex-soldier*

I jumped at the opportunity ODA gave me within a year of my report: to return on a visit and find suitable health sector projects for the UK Government to fund. So back I went in 1990, for ODA/DFID for a short stay under less monitored and restrictive conditions. I visited the major UN agencies out there, as well as the British NGOs (Oxfam, SCF and some Christian agencies). Some of them had been working for more than five years under very difficult conditions and they were not allowed outside Phnom Penh for fear of mines and hold-ups. Their foreign staff had to live in the only open hotel – the *Samaki* or *Royal* – and they had their offices in the same place. I met UNICEF and WHO representatives and saw their programmes, including UNICEF's impressive one for child health, especially the vaccination of the entire unimmunised child population. I succeeded in getting large contributions from ODA for this programme.

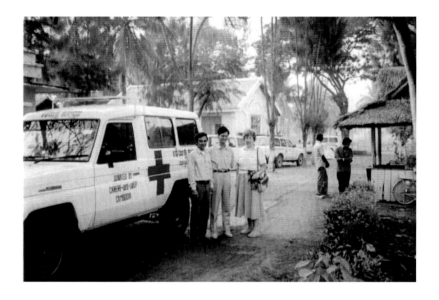

*Visiting a renovated hospital in the war zone*

All UN agencies were having a difficult time because of the travel restrictions. Cambodia had not been accepted into the UN family of nations, and they did not have a democratically elected government. The Cambodia People's Party (CPP) effectively governed the country, except for a few places near the Thai border, so the UN agreed to help to run elections and, in the interim, to govern most of Cambodia fairly effectively. The UN Transitional Authority for Cambodia (UNTAC) was born and UN soldiers arrived to make – and keep – the peace. Troops came in from USA, France, UK, Thailand, India, China, Vietnam and later, Ghana, Nigeria and Algeria.

However, that was after I had gone back to Cambodia on transfer from

ODA to the WHO. I had met up with the local representative of WHO, Dr Brian Doberstyn, who was enthusiastic to re-establish the health services and to establish an efficient leadership in the Ministry of Health. This struck an immediate chord with me and together we worked up a job description and project for a technical adviser to help write the first health plan, to teach health planning and to establish a health planning unit. MOH leaders were keen. Then I had to go home, get the project agreed and funded and, above all, to volunteer myself for the position, including being seconded from ODA to WHO, which I managed, with help from colleagues, for a limited two-year period. There began the most fascinating assignment of my career, lasting from 1992 to 1994.

# Chapter 10: Cambodia III:  Phnom Penh 1992-1994

## World Health Organisation Cambodia 1992

Returning to live in Phnom Penh was mentally stressful for me.  I received huge support from Kan and her husband Huot; also from another previous World Vision staff member, Noing Pak Heang, a construction engineer.  His 17-year-old daughter, Lina, was a good shopper and translator, who has remained a good friend since.  Her father and mother had a bad war and emerged very traumatised, so much so that Pak Heang would not come from his house to meet me for three months; he was too frightened of foreigners and what might happen to him if he was seen talking to me.  Incidents like this were all too common and I had a lot to learn about the trauma and hate that had been engendered by the war.

## New initiatives

I soon found myself a small flat to rent and quickly started work at the WHO office in town.  Dr Brian took me to meet the Ministry of Health and especially my counterpart, Pharmacist Seng Lim Neou, Director of the new Planning Unit.  I came to know the Ministry of Health very well, though at first it was unfriendly.  Eyes followed me closely as I walked up the two flights to the second floor.  Who on earth was this strange new foreigner?  I met the Minister, Dr Chea Tang, and the senior executive, Dr Mam Bun Heng, who became a great friend.  (Note: he has just, as I write this in 2008, become the Minister of Health.  I am proud of him.)  The first thing the Minister said to me was, 'We want you to speak English to us all the time. Don't speak French or Khmer.  Please help us.'  He spoke in fluent French but never did progress much in English.  Seng Lim Neou was a fanatical student, both of English and health planning.  We shared an office and when I went to work around 7.00 am (we made an early start there) he was always in the office with book and headphones, learning grammar.  Of course I tried to help him.  Now he is a very senior senator in his government, where he no doubt uses his good English to advantage.

## Language

The language issue was emotive. The second language which the majority of public servants spoke fluently was French. France provided a huge amount of assistance to rebuilding Cambodia in those early years and their programmes were often conditional on French remaining the accepted second language, for instance in the medical school. (Indeed, medical students were taught in French until 2005, when English became the language used.)

However, the new leadership, the Cambodia People's Party (CPP), had other ideas. They found themselves disadvantaged at international meetings and when receiving important delegations from the USA, UK and Japan. Now they wanted to speak English at the top levels. Many of them worked very hard to learn. When I started work at the Ministry of Health, I was asked to speak English all the time – no French please, and certainly no Khmer. My French was quite tolerable then; not so my Khmer. I had learnt a good deal of Khmer from my interpreters, Thivan and Kan, back in World Vision days, but they once made me promise not to speak Khmer at meetings or to any senior Khmer people. They explained that the Khmer I spoke was strictly for conversing with people of low status (i.e., refugees) and certainly not Ministers or senior doctors. They insisted this would reflect very adversely on them. I complied as I did not want to offend. Anyway, it helped enormously that I could understand Khmer fairly well, though sometimes it caught my colleagues out when I entered discussions!

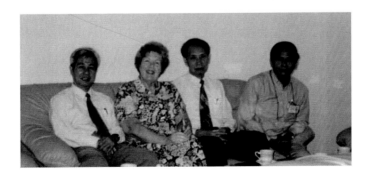

*Seng Lim Neou, me, Chea Thang, Ke Tuy Seang*

What was our job? We were to write a Health Plan for all Cambodia. Neou said he was told that he had just three months to finish a draft in Khmer and that he must do it or lose his job! I was there to show him how. There was nothing to go on; no previous Plan; no health statistics; no maps of hospitals and clinics; no staff lists. We did not know how many nurses and doctors existed or where they were. Communications were very limited; phones did not work. We had to physically go to the places to find out anything – until we could get systems up and running.

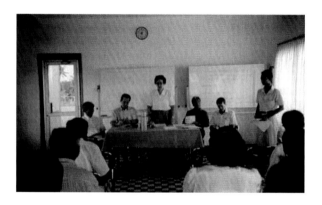

*Teaching at a Health Plan consultation*

## Quick Impact Projects

Very quickly I instilled into my colleagues that any plan had to be based on what was there now – that was the starting place. But no one knew what there was. Then I was asked to join a large and exciting United Nations Development Programme (UNDP) to go out into the provinces to establish what *was* there and what the most urgent needs were. This was the beginning of the QIPs.

One objective of this exploratory mission was to find good projects that were really needed and would quickly impact on people's lives. The amount of money for each project was limited, so, for example, I could not propose complete renovation of a district hospital, but I could and did propose new equipment such as X-ray machines and operating-table instruments. I could include simple health centres/clinics and those were high on my list of

226

priorities, with the serious limitation of a lack of staff to run them.

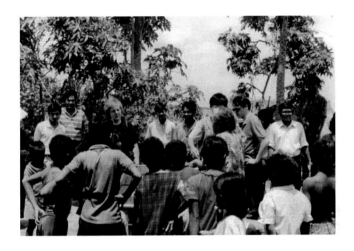

*Village visit – looking at health situation*

I know we included a project to set up and equip nurse and midwife training schools in the provinces. We travelled everywhere in convoys, with UN flags and escorts. Unexploded mines were the great hazard on the roads; and if we stopped, woe betide any silly person who went off-road for any reason; road verges had been favourite places for laying mines.

We were also permitted to propose partnering NGOs who were doing good work but were short of funds. Rehabilitation workshops and limb-fitter came into this. All the baseline information that I collected on a town was of immense value to me as I started work with my counterpart, Seng Lim Neou.

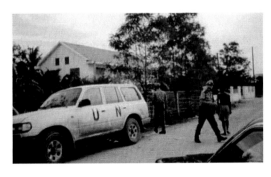

*My UN transport*

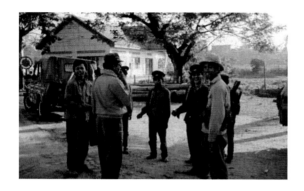

*Our body guards*

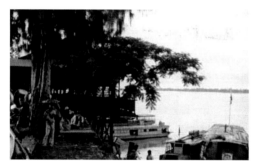

*Kratie Wharf*

*Kratie Province*
*– 'our' boat*

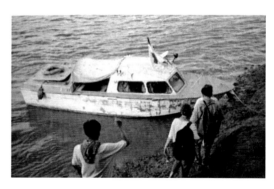

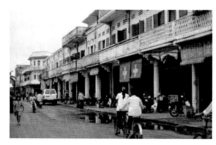

*Kratie Town –*
*10 Pharmacies !*

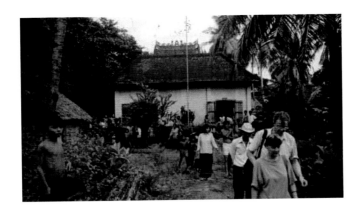

*Commune Infirmary in a Pagoda –Kratie district*

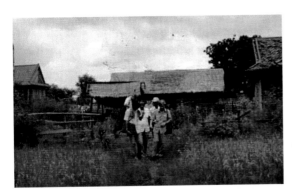

*Commune Infirmary*

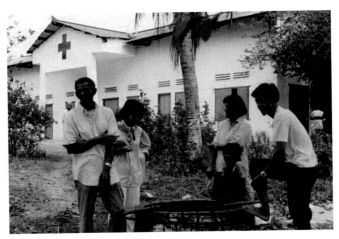

*Examining the old well at Preah Net Preah District Hospital*

229

*Chhlong District Hospital*
*– well and latrine*

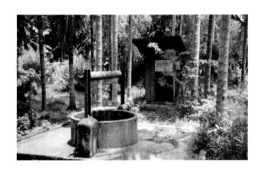

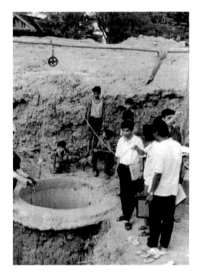

*A new well, 1993*

We visited district hospitals, health centres and two regional hospitals up-country. We stayed in very poor accommodation. There were no hotels open then; we just went where the local chiefs could find a place to put us. Some were very dirty and cockroaches abounded; water was scarce and showers not available. I recall one real 'black hole' in a tenement building in Battambang town. I believe it used to be a school hostel. Cockroaches were everywhere – and rats. I could not sleep at all. The food was not bad, however, as Cambodians are fussy about their food and appreciate good quality rice and fish and dislike poorly cooked food. The best places were the village houses. Fruit was everywhere – delicious mangoes and sacks full of sweet oranges. Our team bumped its way along the pot-holed roads very slowly in a convoy of UN-flagged 4WD vehicles. Many bridges were broken and we forded rivers often.

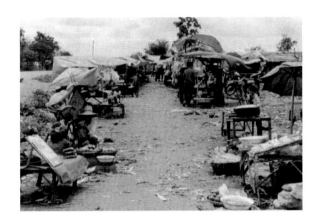

*Road-side stalls*

It was up-country here that we came into contact on the Thai border with the alternative political parties, SON SANN and FUNCINPEC (a French acronym for the 'National United Front for a Neutral, Peaceful And Cooperative Cambodia', which was the royalist party, supported widely by the international community, notably the USA, but also Britain and France). My brief was to advise and assist all the parties. Though I was based in the so-called Ministry of Health in Phnom Penh, in reality it did not have any government remit and was an arm of the Cambodia People's Party (CPP) – led by Hun Sen, and managing around 70% of the country and people. So next I had to help FUNCINPEC to develop a health plan and health services for the whole country. Their health officers had little experience and did not know Cambodia, having all been out of the country for years. Some had been working in the Thai border camps, where many international organisations had been very active in training health workers and building health services for the thousands of refugees from Cambodia.

I had a memorable visit to the northwest before the election. In WHO, we were trying to bring the factions together to pave the way for the health service after the election. At that time, each faction was running its piece of the country, including the health service. One result was that the health forces were all different. There were doctors trained in many ways. FUNCINPEC had many doctors who were western-trained (mostly in France), while the Khmer Rouge had Chinese-trained medics. How would they relate to the State of Cambodia doctors, few though there were? Then a new, more urgent issue arose. The State of Cambodia was implementing the recommended WHO immunisation programme for all the children. It was the normal one in use world wide. But FUNCINPEC was using a different programme of vaccines, funded by USAID.

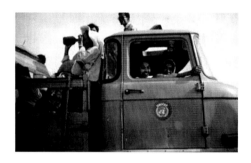

*UNICEF Food Truck*

We badly wanted to bring them together and standardise immunisations countrywide. WHO had already started up joint meetings of the senior medical people from each faction, except that the Khmer Rouge had never come to these meetings. We had no idea what they were doing, so when an opportunity arose to hold a meeting near the Thai border, close to the Khmer Rouge headquarters, I called for the meeting to be held under UN auspices, on neutral ground at the UNTAC camp. My State of Cambodia Ministry team were not keen and did not understand why we needed such a meeting, but we went ahead and the FUNCINPEC and SON SANN medical advisers turned up. We had arranged for the International Red Cross to escort the fearful Khmer Rouge doctors to the meeting, and it worked. I knew all the representatives except the Khmer Rouge, who I knew had trained in Cambodia pre-war, but the doctors, who were late, were all extremely nervous. Without my presence this would not have gone ahead.

I was asked to chair the meeting, being a neutral outsider and representing WHO. The first decision was what language we should use. The CPP delegate could speak English and French; the FUNCINPEC Delegate only French; the KR delegate only Khmer. Of course they could all speak Khmer – but would not admit it. I was prepared to conduct the meeting in Khmer with translation. I had an English-speaking Khmer doctor sitting beside me. But no, it seemed to be a point of honour that the meeting not be held in Khmer. So we struggled along in English, with all delegates having difficulty understanding me or each other. It was so stupid. I decided to make the agenda entirely technical and try not to get political at all. We started with the immunisation schedule and moved on to health worker comparisons, but they really struggled, as did I. I called a break and went off to find a 'rest room' in the camp. I was away about 20 minutes, spinning it out to see if they could get anywhere without me. To my delight, when I went back, they were all chattering away to each other in Khmer. They told me they had all been at medical school together before the war, so knew each other well! I stepped down as chair and Mam Bun Heng and Chun Ly swept through the agenda at speed and with mutual goodwill.

I tried hard to understand why they had been so fearful. I found it hard to understand why they were all so nervous. We were all just doctors: surely we could understand each other. One of them said to me, 'If you had experienced the senseless brutality of the KR you might understand.' All of them had lost relatives, some had lost wives and children, to the KR. They told me it was laughable to consider the KR developing health services for Cambodia. All they could do was to destroy. Of course I don't know what they said to each other but they departed cordially and seemed no longer afraid. We continued with the meetings up to the election and beyond, but we wrestled with the issues of health worker comparability for a long time – and they still do. Perhaps because no one is paid well, it does not matter if you are officially a doctor or just a medical assistant – the work is much the same in the rural clinics.

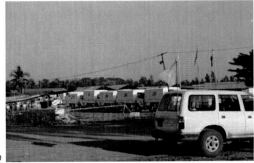

*Sisophon UNTAC Camp*

I remember a very high-level and important Japanese delegation to the Ministry of Health. The Japanese gave millions of dollars to Cambodia then,

233

but certainly did not speak French. They brought a French/Khmer interpreter with them. This poor man placed himself alongside the Secretary of State for Health, Dr Mam Bun Heng, who by now spoke quite good English, but better French. He pretended he could not understand French and asked to speak English. I had come to the meeting late and could not understand what was going on with my Cambodian colleagues, who could certainly understand the French. I started to say so and received a sharp kick under the table from Heng, followed by a wink; I soon caught on to what they were up to and I explained afterwards to the friendly Japanese that my colleagues really did understand and speak English – though not Japanese – and that they wanted very much to be seen as well-educated, English-speaking people. The Japanese delegation were much amused by the explanation and they apologised to the Cambodians for presuming to bring along a French interpreter, not an English one. I think they thought more of Heng through this incident.

Dr Mam Bun Heng and I both wanted the precarious health situation in Cambodia to be known throughout the world. I racked my brains and then concluded that we should together prepare a paper describing the situation in some detail and submit it to medical journals for publications. What I wrote, with Heng, is reproduced in the Appendix as it was – to my delight and pride – published in the British Medical Journal.

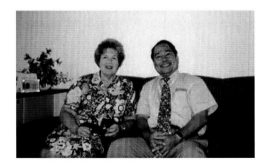

*Myself with Mam Bun Heng, now Minister of Health*

See Appendix 1:

**Cambodian health in transition** by Mam Bun Heng, P J Key
Reprinted from the **BMJ,** 12th August 1995, Vol. 311, Pages 435-437

# NGO Collaboration – The COCOM

Many health NGOs and UN agencies had projects and programmes – sometimes spread country-wide, but more often focusing on provinces nearer to the centres of large towns with good roads. Thus too much assistance went to provinces like Battambang and Kampong Cham, while the poorest and more remote provinces like Ratanakiri, Mondolkire and Preah Vihear got almost no aid.

MOH was in a quandary as to how to manage the distribution of aid better. They knew they needed all the help they could get, so they never refused anyone who came to give something, but they did want to be more in control of what and where. There was a legendary day when a young German doctor arrived in the Minister's office with a case full of dollar bills and announced he was a paediatrician and that he intended to build and run a children's hospital in Phnom Penh. He just wanted permission and land. Dr Chhea Tang accepted gratefully, without considering important questions like staffing and running costs; he could not offer land but agreed to facilitate a meeting with the King, who could give land, which he duly did. This project upset World Vision greatly as they had just built and handed over to MOH the new National Children's Hospital.

Dr Beat Richner has stayed ever since. He is a fine cellist and entertainer. He raises money for his work by concerts back home as well as from visiting tourists locally. He now fully supports two children's hospitals in Phnom Penh and one in Siem Reap. He and his teams of expatriate staff have undoubtedly saved more young Cambodian lives than any other people, NGOs or agencies.

Back in the MOH in 1992 we met often to discuss how better to coordinate aid, to be spread more fairly. Mam Bun Heng came up with the best idea which we followed. He established the 'Coordinating Committee for Health of MOH' (COCOM), which still exists. The Minister himself or his deputy (usually Mam Bun Heng) chaired regular meetings. The Secretariat was the Planning Unit, who prepared Agendas and acted as an executive to the COCOM. So Seng Lim Neou and I set about making COCOM work. Before we started we sent questionnaires to all the outside agencies who wanted to be involved. They already had their own coordinating body, called the MEDICAM, so they decided they would elect their representatives to the COCOM and would collaborate with MOH in this new venture. Most agencies were keen to collaborate – that is, until they were summoned to the Planning Unit to present their proposed programmes and seek approval from us and the COCOM.

We wrote Terms of Reference for COCOM and its Secretariat, which have developed over the years. The big organisations like WHO, UNICEF and the IFRC were automatically members and their assistance was vital to the MOH at that time. I am pleased to say that it was a success. In retrospect this was one of my most important contributions to the MOH at that time. I introduced similar structures in other Ministries of Health in other countries where I worked (Albania and Kosovo).

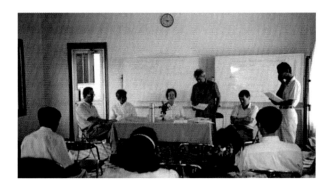

*Management Seminar 1992*

Another problem to us then was the health of the UN soldiers and other expatriate workers. They were living in poor conditions, often tented camps in remote malaria areas; and they contracted and even died from the disease which was becoming resistant to the usual drugs. They also regularly went down with typhoid and dengue fever. What MOH had to do was set up a surveillance system countrywide to map the disease outbreaks and inform the army medical teams of the dangers. Each army contingent brought their own medical team, but they were not all well-informed about tropical diseases and one of WHO's tasks was to set up training for army doctors and army laboratory staff to update and inform them about standard treatments. Even the Australian teams had never seen malaria parasites and did not

236

know how to treat dengue fever. Gradually the UNTAC panic calmed down and incomers were better informed and more careful.

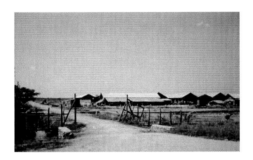

*UN Transit Centre 1992*

We were extremely busy in the MOH Planning Unit at that time. We had to prioritise tasks, which itself was a learning process for the staff. They were used only to doing what they were told and were not used to working things out for themselves or questioning their seniors.

I was involved in a lot of consultations about the three-month health plan of the CPP. We held our first workshop consultation with all the provincial and hospital directors to discuss the Plan. I can still see this group now. It fell to me to introduce the Plan and give out simple questions to groups for discussion and response. We divided them up and asked them to start. 'Any questions?' I asked. An elderly hospital director stood up and asked for explanation. He asked, 'Do you mean you are asking our opinion? We are never asked what we think – do you really want to know this?' What a wonderful lesson this was to me and my staff. It led me to realise the uphill struggle we would have to develop a plan owned by the whole of MOH, but it did help me to understand what oppression they had all suffered and to wonder how best to get their help and advice. We completed this three-month emergency health plan around June 1993. It went for debate to CPP functionaries and was passed by Hun Sen himself. It was printed in Khmer script and English.

My second job at that time (1992-4) was to work with and for WHO. I was expected to feed in to other staff what MOH was doing and planning. WHO then had advisers in malaria, immunisation, medical education, human resource development, and nursing. Most of them collaborated very well and were keen to be part of the planning process. I made good friends among them. Because I was first in the office, I was automatically appointed deputy to the WHO Representative (the boss) in his absences. I found this difficult and it really stopped my MOH work as he was away a lot at conferences in Manila or Geneva.

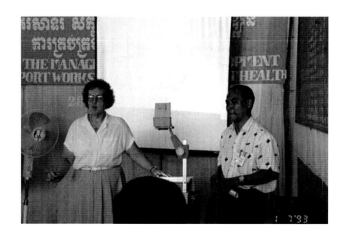

*Kandal Workshop June 1993*

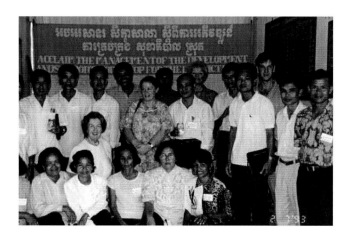

These were anxious days with so many staff, both expatriate and local, travelling extensively through the country. There were armed hold-ups of vehicles – usually by Khmer Rouge soldiers but sometimes by demobbed government soldiers. They would stop the vehicle at gunpoint, force the driver and passengers out, make them strip of all clothing and then drive the vehicle away, leaving the victims to fend for themselves. Vehicles were in high demand. Many NGOs lost them this way. One Japanese volunteer lost both his vehicle and his life. We had Land Cruisers stolen from our locked compound in Phnom Penh one night. Our guards were tied up and locked up – I found them next morning. As acting-in-charge, I had to take responsibility for what all staff were doing and where they were going. It was not easy to continue with my MOH job under these circumstances.

## UN Election

Election day dawned. I was recruited as an observer of the count. The electoral process was monitored closely by teams from outside, e.g. European Union, SADAC, ASEAN and USA. I visited lots of polling stations in villages and towns to get the flavour of the day among the people. It was a public holiday and their first-ever general election. The mood of excitement was everywhere evident. Of course money changed hands in return for votes and chiefs tried to make people vote as they told them; but as far as I could see myself, there was no overt pressure at the polling station. Voting was very private and no one could see how a person voted.

That night it was my job to go to the huge UN warehouse, converted into a vast hall for counting. Teams of Cambodians had been taught how to count and UN officials were everywhere watching and supervising. I saw many of my Cambodian friends there, from all parties. Most MOH staff were CPP supporters and many had party posts and were also observing the count for their party. It was fun and we all had a good time. When we left at dawn, all boxes received had been counted but boxes from remote places were awaited. They were brought in by UN helicopters later. Excitement was mounting but results would not be made known until next evening after more UN and observer scrutiny.

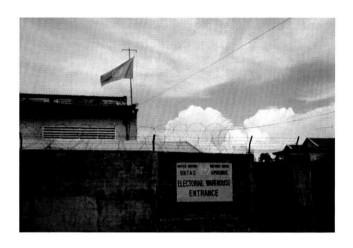

*Phnom Penh UNTAC*

In the evening the whole city population converged along the riverside, where huge boards had been erected to post results when they came that evening. The crowd was vast but we put up our UN flag and got near enough to see the writing. To much surprise, FUNCINPEC won by a small margin. Other parties were way outside. FUNCINPEC, the royalist party, was led by the King's son, Prince Rannaridh, who had been exiled in France. People I knew and worked with were very upset and they still say that the UN rigged the election as they wanted a change from CPP. The results were very close and it seemed that Hun Sen was not ready to concede the result. He demanded a coalition government and to be Prime Minister himself.

It took months to sort out the mess. The UN accepted a coalition and agreed for two Prime Ministers: Ranaridh to be first PM, and Hun Sen second PM. Ministerial posts were to be shared out between the parties. I was not happy to learn that both Health and Education portfolios were taken by FUNCINPEC. This meant big changes and a fresh start to planning for the new Minister in charge. Hong Sun Huot, a French exile, was appointed Minister and Chea Tang retired. Mam Bun Heng's post remained and he hung on. Several completely new FUNCINPEC top officials were brought in. They were almost all French-speaking and orientated to French medicine and organisation. They had no concept of primary health care and were more interested in developing hospitals than health centres. The new minister was more understanding. He had worked

240

with USAID and even with me during the previous year and he did understand what we were wanting him to do. He worked very hard at that time, spending long hours in the ministry. He held early morning staff meetings for all heads of department and I was privileged to be invited to attend them, but he would not hold them in any language but Khmer; I was to follow Khmer or not come. So I did. I had a system: a good friend sat next to me and at a sign from me he would murmur the meaning or even write something down for me. It was a steep learning curve for me and I was proud to be able sometimes to offer help or advice.

Our Planning Unit was given department status and a higher profile. We were tasked to produce a new Five-year Health Plan with budget, all using the FUNCINPEC manifesto, which I had helped write.

The new minister travelled out and about a lot. He really wanted to see for himself what the problems were in the public health service. I often went with him and found him receptive to WHO policies and programmes. He was not medically trained himself so needed a lot of help to understand the hospitals and their problems. He was just horrified at what he found, as I had been previously. But he had almost no money to share out. The country just did not have money for public services. Salaries remained painfully low and many good staff defected to work with NGOs and international agencies, who offered better salaries and training opportunities.

My time to leave grew closer; I had been there two years (my contract time). Much as I wanted to stay, and I believe MOH wanted me, too, I needed to be at home for my ailing mother, as well as for my post at ODA. I was not well; I had increasing pain in one hip and was very disabled, finding walking difficult.

I was able to secure my WHO post for continued ODA funding and then to hand over personally to my successor, Julian, as Planning Adviser to MOH.

I had a memorable send-off from Cambodia Ministry of Health (MOH) and WHO. MOH hosted a wonderful dinner party for me with the present and previous Ministers. I shall never forget the love they showed me as they expressed their gratitude for my contribution. Dr Chea Tang said in a speech, 'You pushed us very hard, sometimes more than we liked, but you made us do it.' I think they all knew I would be back sometime – *I* knew that this was not the last goodbye, as I was to remain ODA's health adviser for Asia, including Cambodia, because of the large funding input we had built up. I would certainly visit regularly to monitor this spend. My heart was there with them all as I left.

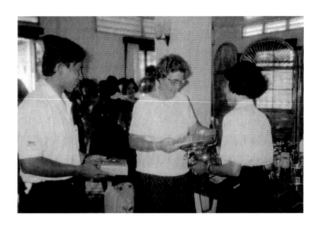

*My farewell party*

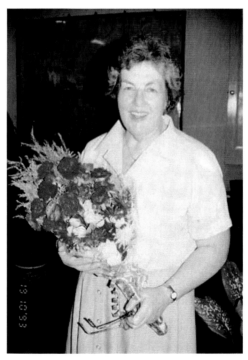

*Flowers from the MOH*

This time it was much harder to leave my 'family'. By this time Kan was really my sister and Huot another brother. I think I was more a grandma than an auntie to their three children John, Kannary and baby Rattana. I was made to feel one of their family, though this put obligations on me too. They were very poor and life was a struggle still. It was hard to say goodbye, but my full intention was to return soon.

*\*\*\**

*Because our two stories had begun to overlap more and more ever since my trip to Cambodia in 1989, I will let Kan tell the rest of her tale here. There will be repetitions in mine later, but her account gives a background of what was happening in this land that was so very dear to me, while I continued my work in many places and countries.*

*\*\*\**

### Kan's story continues

Working with the MOH, I had the chance to go abroad twice; Huot had the chance to go abroad five or six times. So we saved pocket money very carefully.

In 1991, I decided to resign from the MOH and changed to work with a non-government organization, the World Council of Churches. I got paid in US dollars and my life improved from that time. Huot also moved to work for the 'Hygiene and Epidemiology Centre'. Huot and I always changed jobs in the same year.

In 1992 the Republic of Cambodia changed to become the State of Cambodia. Meetings were organised in Peking and Paris between HE Hun Sen and King Norodom Sihanouk to solve the peace problem. The meetings established the Supreme National Council to arrange for the United Nations to work for an election. This was UNTAC (United Nations Transitional Authority for Cambodia) and UNTAC members from many countries occupied Cambodia everywhere, from the city to all the countryside. During that time people improved their businesses well. Houses and land benefited from renting or selling at a good price.

Dr Pene came back to Cambodia working for the MOH, funded by World Health Organization. My family became very close to her and the relationship was as a family, sister and brother. We looked after each other and visited every week, taking good care.

I changed my work to Voluntary Services Overseas (VSO) and Huot changed to work for the Cambodian Red Cross. We knew many people from the different ranks, both Cambodian and foreigners. Dr Tim and Liz Anderson, VSOs, were very good friends to us. I had my last son on December 24th 1992, named Huot Kanrattana Tim. He was delivered by Dr Tim Anderson in the old 7th January Hospital. Before the baby was due, sister Pene collected me, John and Kannary to stay at her house, so Huot was by himself looking after our house.

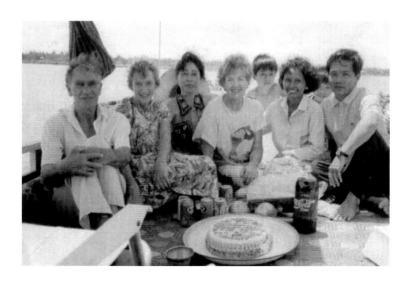

*Dr Pene's birthday party,*
*with Dr and Mrs Anderson, Huot and my family*

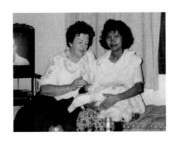

*Dr Pene with Kan and baby Kanrattana Tim 1993*

I celebrated the New Year 1993 at sister Pene's house with Dr Tim and Liz Anderson. We toasted a glass of red or white wine to each other for health, friendship, solidarity and happiness. With the three kids, I went to our new home on January 7th which was a public holiday of remembrance for the revolution date. We had sold the flat opposite MOH and built up a new house at Tuk Laok II District, Khan Tuol Kork. We had saved the money and since August 1991 bought the land from a friend, at a very good price.

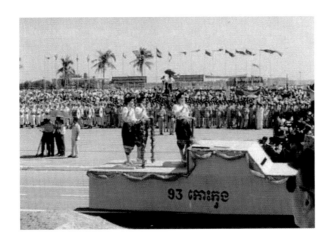

*1993 Cambodia Independence Parade*

In mid-1993, I resigned from VSO to look after the construction of our new house and my baby. I extended the house with two floors –

245

ground floor and first floor. I made eight bedrooms, kitchen, storeroom and garage. After six months of uncertainty following the election, Cambodia settled the results in July 1993. People were very pleased to choose their own party that they liked best and trusted. HE Hun Sen was elected Prime Minister; he was our hero – he had delivered us from the Khmer Rouge.

Luckily, I stayed home only three months. I was called by the Cambodian-British Centre for British teachers to work in their administration office. I enjoyed working with British people very much and I liked my job as well.

In 1994 sister Pene left us when she finished her WHO contract. Also my sister Ratha and her son Sokunthearo were leaving us to live at her own home in Psa Chas. Chhun's mother (Huot's sister) replaced Ratha. She did housework for me and I had one girl to look after baby Tim.

In 1997 we bought two plots of land in Siem Reap as a good investment. We thought about our retirement because we would not receive any pension, so we planned to live or make a business there. We planned and dreamed to build up a guesthouse as a family-run business. I showed these plots of land to many friends for sale or investment, but no one was interested.

In 1998 Chhun, my nephew, finished study at the Faculty of Medicine. He had to go to work at Preah Vihear Province, far away. In 1999, Chanry, my niece, was married to a teacher after she finished her teacher training at the regional centre. Then three months later, Chanry with new husband and her mother left us.

In 2001 Chhun married Nak. We paid for all their (Chhun's and Chanry's) wedding parties as was the custom.

In 2002 my work finished after a two-year contract. I did not want to work any more. The family needed me and I thought I would have enough to do. I had to stay home every morning; I went to the market for food, cleaned the house, cooked and did some crochet work.

Sister Pene often came to work in Cambodia. Every time she visited, she saw I was staying home and was miserable. She asked me how I was feeling. I told her what I had planned in my dream, but my budget was short. Sister Pene organised a visit for me to England with her in February 2002. The objective for that visit to UK was as a holiday, to find out more about colleges and universities for children, and to see old friends: Boran and Sadin Moeun; Charya and Saroeuy Long; Jane Fowles; Pauline Shard; Tim and Liz Anderson. Sister Pene celebrated her birthday and invited her brother, sister-in-law, cousin and husband, relatives and close friends. Then she asked me to write my story under Khmer Rouge, but I could not do it, because it was so cold I could not concentrate on any words. I visited many places with sister Pene and searched for an English cooking book, crochet book, dress-making book and some souvenirs for friends and family in Cambodia.

Then I went to France with Boran and Sadin Moeun for a school reunion in Paris. We were together staying at Mavida's house and the reunion was held at her house too. There were about forty friends invited and two teachers. They brought food from their homes to share with each other. We had plenty of food, beer, wine, champagne, dessert, fruit, cake and biscuits. We had jokes, fun, laughter; we were so excited about each memory and I was interested and enjoyed it.

By chance, I had a phone call from the two cousins in Lyon; they asked me to visit them. They paid for a round trip ticket on the High Speed Train for me. We had lost contact since 1974, so after they heard that I was in Paris, I had to stay one night with Siri Penn and another night with Sujani Penn, Jean-Pierre (husband) and Cecilia, whose daughter is the same age as John.

It was such a wonderful visit: exciting, enjoyable, pleasant and especially very delightful. Throughout the darkness of blood and fear,

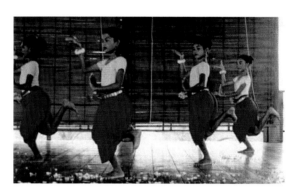

*Girls performing a traditional dance*

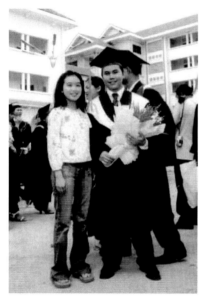

*John and Kannary at his graduation*

John graduated from the National University of Management. He would have liked to carry on to a Master's degree. Kannary studied in three places: the University of Science and Information Technology, the University of Panasatra, and language at the Australian Centre for Education. Rattana Tim studied at Santhor Mok Primary School We love the three children very much and they listen to us as well.

***

Sister Pene was very good to my family. She knew us very well now and she discussed with us what would happen in the future if I did not have a job. So she made a plan with us to visit our land in Siem Reap. We went by plane because the road was bad in March 2002. Pene, Huot, Kan and Tim left Phnom Penh on Friday night's last flight to Siem Reap. We saw both plots of land: one was 30m x 60m (= 1,800 square metres) and I had already made a concrete fence around the whole area, and the other was in a rice field 45m x 40m (= 1,800 square metres) without a fence. After we made a study, we made a business visit to a hotel, a guesthouse, a restaurant, the market and the Temple. We returned to Phnom Penh on Monday morning with the early flight.

This visit was very important to us and we could see there would soon be light in our life. Then we had a family meeting. Huot showed us his design for the land; we discussed whether we could make a right decision on it and made an agreement to start our project. John and I would stay on the land all the time, making a business.

From November 2002, John and I packed our luggage to go to live in Siem Reap. We rented a house from the neighbour opposite our land to watch the construction work and we were always there from then on, watching the construction project. Huot, Kannary and Tim lived in Phnom Penh. We met each other once a month but we talked by phone every day. Sister Pene went to visit the project twice that year. The building was finished in November and we put equipment and furniture in later. I found a school for Tim so he moved to study in Siem Reap. Huot and Kannary were still in Phnom Penh. In December, sister Pene came to celebrate Tim's birthday on 24th and on January 1st we celebrated the guesthouse warming party. We employed a guard, cleaners, cook and John as the General Manager. We had many guests and tourists checking in and out and we were very busy from January 2004. Time flew very quickly and a year passed with the business running well.

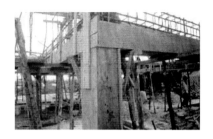

*Damnak Chan*
*– early construction*
*and below, nearing completion*

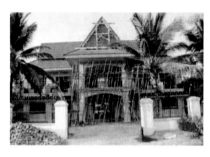

*Family at the back of*
*the new guesthouse,*
*2004*

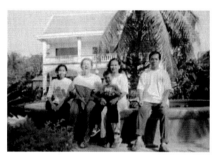

Early in the year 2005, sister Pene travelled to work in Cambodia; as usual she came twice and planned to come again in September, but unluckily her health became a problem in August. Sister Pene had a stroke and fell down in the garden at her house. Her neighbour saw and called the hospital. Her cousin Peggy sent an email to us but we were very worried. We prayed to God to make her recover soon. We loved and missed her very much. I emailed to Boran and Sadin Moeun to visit her for me, and they told me sister Pene wanted me to come, but not until the doctor allowed her back home. Now we had difficulty with communication because sister Pene could use only her right hand as her left hand was useless.

In 2006 she wrote a letter to Huot, Kan and Kannary to invite us to visit her in the United Kingdom for three months from March. We were very pleased to visit her; I would have liked to stay with her longer to look after her in her illness, but she preferred Kannary to stay longer – for six months. And I should go back to look after the guesthouse and Huot needed to get back to his work. We arrived at her house very late at night. Ms Patricia, her carer, came to welcome us and show us our bedroom. She said sister Pene would see us for breakfast next morning. Sister Pene appeared to meet us in an electric wheelchair; she smiled to us; her white face looked bright but there were signs of tiredness. Patricia arranged her breakfast: cereals of different kinds, yoghurt, milk, orange, banana, orange juice, coffee, and a box of weekly medicine. I had brought some mangoes for her and I cut one for her breakfast every morning; that's her favourite fruit, too. I cooked Cambodian food for her and gave massage. Huot helped me to cook and chat with her. Kannary helped with some computer work and massaged her Auntie. Sister Pene made a plan of visits all the time to entertain us. Finally, she wanted to come to Siem Reap again in December for two months. She had thought about the business and she provided funds to establish a swimming pool in the guesthouse to make more income. In April, Huot and I left sister Pene but Kannary stayed to be there with Auntie until the end of August.

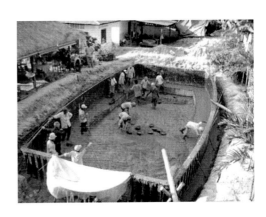

*Construction of the pool*

253

*And a further note by Pene:*

*After I retired in 1998, I was able to obtain work with WHO or NGOs so that I could pay annual, or even biannual, visits to Kan and her family. This enabled me to be closely involved with them as they set about the difficult job of providing an income to start their three children in the world...*

But let me go back to the time that I was to leave Cambodia in 1992, when Kan and Huot were facing financial hardship. They just had to find a way to support themselves and their family in their old age. There are no pensions in Cambodia. We had many discussions, especially about the children's education. I promised to keep in touch and to help them in any way I could. They had done so much for me.

Soon after I left, Kan retired from her job and stayed at home all day looking after her little boy, Rattana Tim, and running the house. But she was very unhappy and bored with her life. On one of my subsequent visits, I felt that she needed serious help for the future and we held the first of several family conferences. I learned what I did not know – that they had some land in the provincial town of Siem Reap. This was exciting. Seam Reap is the tourist town for the famous Angkor Wat temple complex and was being developed fast by government as a tourist centre. I felt that there could be possibilities for their future involvement in a business in Siem Reap. So we visited together over a long weekend. I had my first sight of Kan's land: the plot, a rectangular walled area behind the airport road, was undeveloped and overlooked by new large hotels. It was big enough to develop and it was all theirs. We stayed overnight in a new guesthouse which was run by a retired policeman with his wife's support and help from a Japanese investor. It gave us all many ideas and was the spur for Huot and Kan to take on a guesthouse as their own business. I undertook to support through limited funding, as I could earn. Huot planned all the building himself; he learned how to produce scale plans on his computer and he designed the building with some advice from an architectural colleague. We all got excited.

During my next visit, a year later, they were ready to put the plans out to a builder to contract; Kan decided to move to live in Siem Reap to oversee the building construction. She rented a room with a neighbour and took young

256

John with her. He had just finished his university course in management and he was keen to be involved in the family business. Together they spent the next year living there and watching the building grow up. Huot visited occasionally to see that all was well. My next visit in December 1998 was to be for the 'grand opening' of the guesthouse. They were anxiously awaiting connections to electricity and telephone. I flew direct to Siem Reap from Bangkok, arriving one evening after dark. The family were all there to meet me, ready to show off their work, and I was to stay in my new home. Then, disaster struck; there was no electricity in the house. The arrangement with a nearby hotel had been cut off, unknown to them. So I went there in the darkness and decided it was no good trying to overnight there in the dark. There was a small guesthouse down the road and I went there and next morning had my first tour of our home for my disappointed family. It was soon sorted out and I moved in with them and we started the next planning phase – it was serious business.

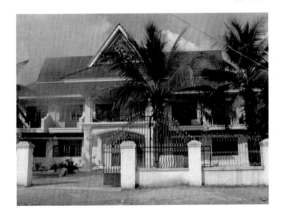

*Our completed guesthouse, Damnak Chan*

We had a building, now we needed to develop the furnishings and prepare publicity such as brochures, advertisements and pictures. I was hooked on it, loving the challenge. It made up for my retirement leisure and made a new outlet for my energy – another project, and continuing my mission to assuage my survivor's guilt. Kan and I toured furniture makers and stores and eventually placed orders for beds, tables, chairs and wardrobes. We planned to open half the rooms to earn money and to extend the fittings to all the rooms as soon as possible. I had my own designated en suite room leading onto the first floor balcony. It was very comfortable, with air conditioning, TV and fridge. I loved it dearly and planned to make long visits every year to help and support my family. Then Kan and I together planned the garden, which had been flooded badly that year. We sought out shrubs and orchids and made an orchid nursery. Kan found the staff – all local women from nearby villages. And we employed a guard to look after security and do some gardening. The staff are given very low salaries. Together they cooked, washed, cleaned and were generally at everyone's beck and call. Kan's son John manned the front desk and generally helped deal with guests and their needs. Meanwhile, Kannary was at college and young Tim was at school in Phnom Penh. He very soon moved to the high school in Siem Reap and became a part of the family there.

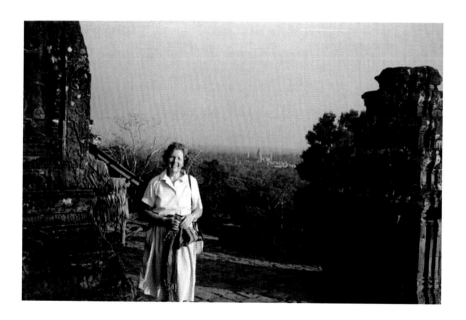

*Myself before the view of Angkor Wat from Phnom Bakeup*

I made visits to them from 2001 up to 2005 at least once a year, always finding consultancy work to do for one organisation or another. In 2004 we finally decided to invest in a private swimming pool in the grounds. This was one of the best things we did. We mostly borrowed the money and are still paying it back. But it has proved its worth over and over again as it is a big attraction to visitors. I became ill in 2005 and had to miss out that year but I was able to return for Christmas 2007, and again in 2008, to find out what was going on.

This has been a great interest for me and has totally absorbed my leisure time, but it has not all been plain sailing. The competition among guesthouses and hotels in Siam Reap is very great. When the tourists do not come, then the business does not do well. We have a good reputation and we even got put into the *Lonely Planet* guide book, which helped fill up the rooms. Very recently (in 2009), Kan and Huot and the family decided to convert the guesthouse into six apartments, which are let out on a long-term basis, mostly to expatriates who go there to work. It is doing quite well like this and is much less work for Kan and the family.

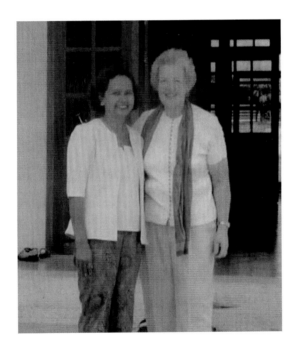

*Kan and Pene, 2005*

# Chapter 11: 1995 Further work with ODA – now DFID London again

On my return from Cambodia in 1994, ODA (Overseas Development Administration) had become DFID (Department for International Development), and from Cambodia, I went back to my previous position in ODA as Principal Health Adviser, but almost immediately, in autumn 1994, had three months' sick leave for a hip replacement operation. I returned to work in early 1995 and was given main responsibility for the ODA's support to health research and for the monitoring of the considerable financial support for the two Schools of Tropical Medicine, London and Liverpool. I remember, during my convalescence, being sent a pile of some thirty health research proposals to read and scrutinise for possible funding. I was glad to do it as my active mind rebelled at my immobility.

Back at work, a bit handicapped but no longer in pain, I took up the reins and limped my way onto my travels again. Then Mother finally died after long years away from us all in her own demented world. For me, my mum died when she stopped recognising me, at least two years before her body gave up. But I had a new challenge. I went to Geneva to a big conference, followed very soon by an extraordinary visit to St Helena. I cannot recommend a sea trip in the stormy Atlantic Ocean for rehabilitation from hip surgery; I was too unsteady, but I managed with a good deal of help.

## St Helena

A review of the health and social services of the colony of St Helena was due. I was asked to go at short notice, mainly because of my past experience of the Atlantic and Caribbean Islands. St Helena was dependent on the UK for a lot of services, including health, education, finance and others. In the main this meant provision of skilled staff – teachers, doctors, laboratory and X-ray technicians and others. DFID was very keen to work towards self-sufficiency in all sectors, especially health. By now there were a number of trained island doctors, dentists, nurses and so on, all trained in the UK at British expense. However, none would return to practise on the island. It was my job to explain why and make suggestions on what actions needed to be taken. I was also to discuss with government how best they could prepare a full health plan and budget for the health service in the coming years.

I flew to Cape Town to board the MV *St Helena* for the eight-day voyage to St Helena. I know I spent many hours in my cabin reading old reports and books to learn more about the island. I knew so little and felt so unprepared.

One fine morning, with a huge swell rolling, the high cliffs of St Helena rose in front of us. We were soon standing off the pier. The Atlantic swell almost never allowed the ship to go close to disembark passengers. There was a landing barge alongside and passengers had to climb down a long ladder and jump onto the rolling barge. I was not yet all that steady on my feet after my hip operation and was very frightened by this procedure. But the alternative was to be hoisted in the cage that was used for stretcher and wheelchair patients or other infirm people. I rebelled at that and took my chance the other way, with success. Transferring onto the stone pier was another test as it was covered in green slimy, slippery seaweed, and again, the manoeuvre was not helped by the persistent swell. We were met and well cared for by health officials and started on our all-too-short visit – we had to return on the next sailing to Cape Town.

St Helena is an amazing place, almost impossible to describe: it consists of massive rocks and steep slopes with villages dotted on the slopes. There is just one town, Jamestown, located in a steep valley running up from the only port. There are only three places on the island where you can get down to the sea and no beaches at all, just massive boulders with huge waves breaking dangerously for anyone near. Jamestown is small, with three hotels and a few shops – mostly selling goods imported from Cape Town. The one island hospital is at the top of Jamestown, very crowded into a crack between cliffs, which are eroding and fall sometimes onto the hospital and houses. The roads are built into the cliff sides and feel very dangerous at first. Cars have to be good to get up and down.

I was given an orientation tour of the hospital, health centres and homes (to see mental health and retarded children). I met all the health staff, including a lot of local nurses and specialist staff (doctors, tutors, lab technician, pharmacist, dentist) from South Africa, England and India. What a cosmopolitan group it was. The administrator, Ivy Ellick, an Islander, was excellent and became a good friend. She had to put up with a lot from her expatriate and local senior staff but she coped well.

All I could do on that short visit was discuss, observe, listen and report back. It was clear that a lot of changes and a plan were needed to provide a health service up to British standards, which was the aim of local government, as well as of the UK government, for a remaining colony. All the residents were by now British citizens and even British law applies there.

So I travelled with my DFID colleagues back to Cape Town, stopping off to visit hospitals and doctors who provided services for St Helena and Tristan da Cunha. Then by air back to London.

## Second Visit to St Helena

As a matter interest here, after I retired I was asked to pay a repeat visit to St Helena, staying longer and helping Ivy and staff to write their health plan. This was really when my health planning days were confirmed. I went by the same route to St Helena via Cape Town, but was to stay there for three weeks and go home via Ascension Island to review the health services there. This time I stayed at an extremely nice guest-farmhouse out of town and well into the high countryside. I was provided with my own car to drive. I was terrified of the narrow, very steep roads and dreaded the single-track road up and down the cliff face to and from Jamestown.

My task was to assist the health officials to develop a five-year health plan and budget. It was a fascinating experience and it would have been easy to write it myself – but that was not the point. So I had meetings with councillors, Islanders at every level, and all the health staff, local and expatriate. No one had any knowledge of how to do it, so I gave many seminars and soon had a small planning group seconded to me. We succeeded and presented it to government officials and councillors just before the boat came in. What a celebration we had – in one of the few eating houses/pubs. (They all served the same: tuna steaks and chips.) I presented the plan and budget to DFID and the FCO on my return. Of course they said it was too expensive, but at least they now knew what was needed to provide the island with a reasonable level of health care. I am told that the plan was well-supported financially but not so well by the health staff who did not continue to support the aims and objectives they had determined.

Stopping at Ascension Island was interesting – my second time there, but the only time I reviewed the health care. It was hugely different from the service on St Helena. Government had plenty of money coming in – from airport landing fees and shipping charges – and good communications with the UK and Europe. Staff were recruited easily on high salaries and excellent accommodation. Everything there revolved round the airport and its services; it was a major refuelling base between Europe and the south and a telecommunications base. I stayed in single quarters on the base and ate in the mess along with most expatriates. The food was disappointing, and everything was run-down. I was very interested to see the birds and wildlife, especially Turtle Beach. I heard many tales of shipwrecked sailors being stranded there in the past and even stories of deaths from cholera – there was evidence of many graves on the beaches. But I was only given a few short days before I climbed into another RAF plane to Brize Norton, back in the UK. Many St Helenians work on Ascension, for better pay and conditions, and this is to the loss of St Helena, which can ill afford to lose these trained staff.

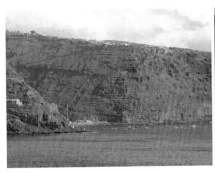 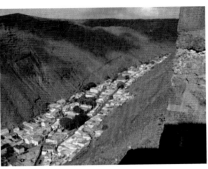

*Approach to Jamestown*          *Jamestown Main Street*

# Sierra Leone

After the first visit to St Helena, I went off to Africa again. ODA had been providing considerable financial and technical support to rebuilding Sierra Leone after the civil war ended in 1995. There was still civil unrest, with rebel groups ranging the country and doing their best to uproot families and inflict horrible wounds on civilians, including young children. Their signature injury was the amputation of limbs – arms, legs and fingers. These poor, suffering people had to treat themselves without the luxury of doctors and hospitals.

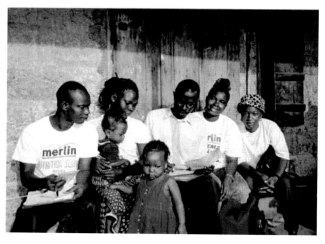

*Sierra Leone –*
*MERLIN and nutrition*
*support*

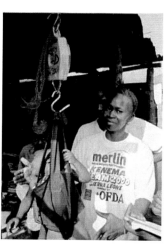

I was sent by ODA with a small team to evaluate the work of several NGOs being funded by ODA, some health programmes and, as well, to discuss health care needs with the very new MOH.

Here was another post-conflict country for me to work with. There was a UN peacekeeping force there providing essential services and facilitating the work of outside agencies and organisations like UNICEF, WHO and UNHCR (UN High Commissioner for Refugees). They ran a helicopter service up-country, known as 'the milk run', on which I hitched a ride to Kenema in the east. (The roads were still too dangerous to travel on, with rebel gangs ready to hold-up, kill, maim and loot. We were not allowed on them.)

The country had been devastated by the war. Buildings in Freetown had been burnt down or shot up. Roads were impassable. I visited the Bishop's house, at the request of the Mission Agency, CMS. There was not much left. Rebels had come in from the sea one night and sacked the fine old Mission House, before burning it. I was given a vivid account by the Bishop and his Archdeacon, who had both witnessed and survived this. The Archdeacon's church in Freetown centre had been burned one night, losing all furniture and furnishings. I saw it later, and was sad.

However, first, I went on a review visit to the NGO MERLIN (Medical Emergency Relief International), which was providing medical relief up-country in Kenema and beyond. They had renovated the district hospital and had set up a huge feeding centre for malnourished children. They had also established mobile medical clinics in the more distant villages. I went out with one and found good work being done by committed local staff under difficult conditions.

One very interesting component of MERLIN's work concerned lassa fever, a rare and fatal virus infection, spread by rats in houses. There had been a lassa fever ward there for several years, being technically supported as a research field unit by USA and UK research centres. I knew little of this dreaded infection before I went there, but learnt a lot on my visit. It was very important that the UN troops were well briefed on it and under constant observation for early signs. A new anti-viral drug had recently become available in China and it offered hope to sufferers if given early. Unfortunately the UN medical teams knew nothing about it and I spent an interesting few hours giving them a full briefing and, essentially, teaching them. They were embarrassed but grateful as they had just heard from the UK that a young man just evacuated by air to a high security infectious disease unit had died on arrival and was diagnosed post mortem as infected by lassa fever virus. They had failed to diagnose his infection, though he fitted all the criteria I had recently learned and he could have been treated and cured if given the new drug.

After Kenema, I was taken to Bo district and town, where there were huge camps of displaced people, fleeing the rebels. Their conditions were bad, with no sanitation or clean water and the inevitable problems among the children. MERLIN wanted to start a new programme in Bo district hospital, to assist government staff to provide an adequate service. It clearly needed funding and I was able to recommend their project to ODA.

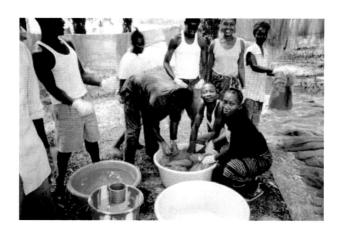

*Sierra Leone – post-conflict health project,*
*impregnating mosquito nets*

I left the country sad and depressed that little long-term help would be given as the base of trained staff was so small and there were no good plans or projects forthcoming. Substantial aid to small African countries was no longer considered worthwhile or a good investment. West Africa was in a real mess then. All I could do was make recommendations and pray that Cambodia did not go down that road. I felt that the future for Sierra Leone was much worse than Cambodia's. The people were very different.

# Chapter 12: Retirement activities

## Retirement, February 1998

After 20 years' service, I left ODA in February 1998, when I had my 60th birthday. I had a memorable send-off from ODA; my office party was large and I was given a lovely farewell present of a cut-glass crystal bowl. As well, I was entertained by medical colleagues at a formal dinner party in a London hotel. I felt very honoured and valued by my big home community.

As I had several weeks' accrued leave, I had decided to take terminal leave and go abroad. I flew off for a wonderful holiday in Australia, where I stayed with my brother John and all his family, as well as old friends from Papua New Guinea. I called in to Phnom Penh on my way to Sydney and was given a wonderful 60th birthday party there by my family, even though it is not customary to celebrate one's birthday in Cambodia. Then I had a fun proper 60th birthday party in Sydney, hosted by my brother and sister-in-law. Many old friends came as well as my Aussie relations.

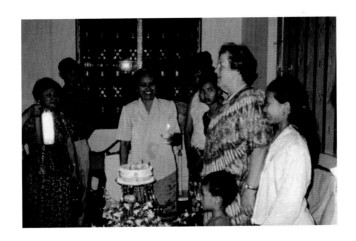

*Making a speech
for my 60th birthday party in Cambodia*

267

I completed my assignment soon after this. I did not want to stay on, as I did not enjoy living in Geneva, finding it lonely and unfriendly, though with excellent living conditions. The contrast to my usual working situation was just too great. Since then, I have watched the progress of the RBM programme with interest. It is really due to this experience that I later helped to found the UK Malaria Consortium.

## Home, Bovey Tracey

And so, from Geneva, back to move into my dear new home, *Hestia*. I loved the house from the start and happily set about re-ordering the lovely garden on the steep hillside. I had a beautiful magnolia tree that bloomed heavily that spring. I was very happy and did not much want to go anywhere again – but that never lasts with me, so I soon set about finding worthwhile occupation close to home. After getting my house straight, I entered fully into the life of my church, calling for more mission outreach and even developing an overseas link with the burnt-out church in Freetown, Sierra Leone.

I gave myself a little time to get settled, but I always knew that I would not just stay put. I felt young and vigorous – partly as a result of having my right hip joint replaced successfully. (It had been giving me trouble since my Cambodia assignment, when it had been aggravated by bumpy roads and an even bumpier boat on the sea.) Also, I had just been invited to go to China to review a project *and* I wanted to return to Cambodia, where Kan and Huot were moving forward well on our new guesthouse venture. But again, my plans were put on hold because of a crisis…

## WHO Albania and Kosovo, 1999

Now, still in 1999, having moved house, I started watching on the TV all the problems in Albania. I had always been fascinated by the stories of that 'closed' – i.e., to foreigners – country, with its people supposedly oppressed by a communist government. I had wanted to go there. Now I got a very

270

strong feeling that my skills were needed there to help the opening-up country to manage the large input of international aid, especially the NGOs. So I was convinced I had another call. After a few phone calls, I found that WHO Emergency Department was seeking someone to go out on a short contract to work in the Albanian Ministry of Health and plan for meeting the needs of both the flood of refugees (from Kosovo) and the local people. I accepted very quickly and was invited to go at once to Copenhagen for discussion of my possible contract. I survived this experience and within two weeks I was on the way to Tirana with a team of United Nations experts. We had had instructions to take just one small suitcase each and to be prepared to carry it. I expected a tour of 3-6 months, so found this a bit difficult. I know I struggled but had to be helped with my overweight bags.

We were made welcome in Tirana and accommodated at a central government hotel in Spartan conditions. I could not believe the scarce food provided, so after presenting myself to the WHO representative, Dr Louis Migliorini, I set about finding a flat to rent. I was helped in this by an NGO, Health Unlimited, of which I was a long-term trustee. I actually took over the rent of a flat they had rented, but no longer needed. It was a second floor flat in central Tirana and was convenient to offices and shops. I soon settled into it, though it was noisy.

In the interim Ministry, I was made welcome, though it became clear that senior officials and the interim Minister had no understanding of what I was supposed to do for them. So I began a task familiar to me and very like my early days with the new government in Cambodia: that of teaching them first. They were keen for my help. The interim Minister was in a complete muddle about all the goods that he was being offered by well-meaning aid agencies. Of course, to him it all sounded too good to be true and he had said yes to everyone until now. He found my lack of enthusiasm for the latest high-tech medical equipment incomprehensible. So I sat down with my small team to create a planning unit from scratch. First we all had to learn and document what people were available, what services existed already, and what was most urgently needed to meet the pressing needs of the refugees.

Albania had an under-developed health service, with a few large hospitals, poorly staffed and badly equipped. Medicines were virtually unobtainable except in the few private pharmacies. The health profile of the groups of people was interesting. Local Albanians had health problems similar to their European neighbours: hypertension, cardiac disease, chest problems, chronic illnesses like diabetes, kidney disease. They were heavy smokers. We did not know the level of infant or child mortality. Children were thin but fairly healthy as far as we could tell. The incoming Kosovo Albanians were less healthy. There were many mental health problems; children had skin diseases and were undernourished; communicable diseases such as measles and whooping cough were spreading in the overcrowded camps and halls. It was clear to me that we needed to plan for the two groups separately; first and most urgently for the refugees, but not excluding the needs of the local people, who clearly had been long neglected.

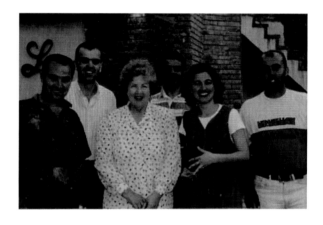

*With the team in Albania, May 1999*

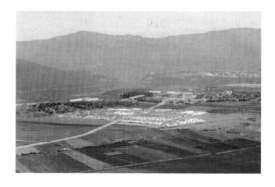

*Refugee camp in Northern Albania, 1999*

272

# WHO Kosovo

By July of that year, 1999, the refugees had mostly streamed back across the border and international focus switched to what was happening in Kosovo, which had taken a beating at the hands of the Serbs and Yugoslavia. Louis Migliorini was transferred from Tirana to head up the new WHO office in Pristina, capital of Kosovo. He kept calling me to persuade me to come out to join him and his team to develop a plan for Kosovo's health services. I weakened after a few weeks. Whether it was the right move for me then I doubt, as I had an unhappy and not very productive time. I flew to Skopje in Macedonia, from where we travelled in a long convoy by road to Pristina. The road was jammed with trucks and returning refugees, the verges mined.

When we reached Pristina town, capital of Kosovo state, we faced two hurdles – somewhere to stay and something to eat. There were no hotels open then, and WHO gave me a local staff member to help me find rented accommodation. There were many empty houses and flats, most locked up and belonging to Kosovos who had left in a hurry without their personal belongings. We simply asked around in the streets and before long were pointed to a flat that had belonged to an elderly couple, who had gone away, no one knew where; but they encouraged me to move in for a few days and leave them some money. So I soon found myself living in a comfortable home, looking after myself in this new environment – a barricaded town with soldiers everywhere on the streets and our movements watched carefully.

Food was the next problem. The shops were empty, by and large, due for replenishment as soon as the trucks got through the blocks. There was no rice, no milk, no vegetables or fruit. There was one Italian restaurant that had set up to feed foreigners, and no doubt to make money out of us; but they only offered pizza or simple pasta; and after a few days of this for every meal, it palls. Gradually conditions improved and by the end of my stay the stores had filled up and the farmers were bringing fruit to sell.

There was an interim, UN-led government for the state; indeed, elections were not held for another eight years, when they took place in 2008. We never quite knew who was in charge; officially it was the UN Special Representative, with a large team of seconded officials from many countries.

275

The local people were scandalised at the newcomers, with their white, UN Land Cruisers and extravagant life styles. Our job was to create and develop systems for every sector: health, education, finance, social welfare, defence, etc. A new police force was recruited and trained by invited expatriate police officers. In the interim the UN Force must keep the peace. The British provided a battalion of marines and I found them rather fierce for this role. I think they would be better in a fighting role. I remember one day having to visit the town centre for medical reasons. The marines had set up road blocks because of a visiting head of state. I mistakenly thought this did not apply to me. How wrong I was. I was brought to a stop in my UN car, faced by a line of fixed bayonets and some fierce marines daring me to try to continue my journey. If *I* was really frightened by them, how much worse it must have been for ordinary Kosovos who knew no English.

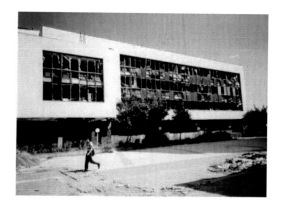

*Kosovo – the burnt-out Ministry of Health, July 1999*

My job here was to establish a small planning cell and, with them, to develop an interim health plan for the Kosovo health services, which were in disarray following the war. The medical and nursing schools had closed and many qualified heath staff, especially doctors, had emigrated to obtain jobs in other European countries. We were starting from a low base and found it particularly hard to find teachers to restart training. Hospitals had been focusing on treatment of trauma, mostly mine injuries but also explosions and bombs. There was a medical school operating at a very low base. I paid an early visit and was quickly besieged with requests for books and journals and any assistance to bring the young students and their teachers up to date. Despite this, there were some excellent doctors in the service, working long hours for a very low wage and with few medicines and poor equipment. This was an urgent need we sought help with right away from the international community. The British aid input was large, through DFID. Their programme focused on rehabilitating the main hospital, providing a surgical team along with equipment and drugs.

I stuck to my rule of assessing the present country situation before starting to plan. My small team with me, I held consultations in every district, with medical, nursing and administrative staff. We drew up a comprehensive report which I presented on WHO's behalf at a UN conference on Kosovo, held in Skopje. It was to provide a starting base and budget for all agencies operating in Kosovo in the health sector. I was then tasked by WHO with developing an interim Health Plan for the state. First I had to identify a suitably skilled team of health professionals, including an economist. It was not easy and was further hampered by the political situation and especially the uncertainty of the UN interim government and their inability to sort out salaries for the public service workforce. There was no pot of money from which salaries could be paid, so few were willing or able to come to work every day with me and my WHO team.

We finished the plan quite quickly and it was time to go home – or stay longer. I did not like Kosovo. It was a state full of hate. There was no love or respect between Serbs and Albanians. The WHO office was not a happy one, lacking in leadership. So we from the UN were stuck in the middle, always trying to mediate but not getting far. It was not possible to progress in developing strong, agreed plans in any sector or to build up the local skills and capacity, without proper living salaries and no firm future support at home. So I handed over to WHO colleagues and gladly sought my own home.

***

After this, it was back to *Hestia* for a while, then to China, West Africa, Cambodia again, and Rwanda...

# Plymouth

Back at my home base in Bovey Tracey, I continued developing more local involvement, but what motivated me most was working in Plymouth to provide support to the influx of asylum seekers and refugees.

I had first met my new African family, the Kallons, in 1991. Sam Kallon was a dear man, a refugee himself from Sierra Leone, where his wife and children had been killed and lost to the rebel insurgents. He was an architect by training and had done further study in Russia – he spoke good Russian.

Although he found life in Britain hard at first, Sam was granted leave to remain in the UK when all Sierra Leoneans were deemed British citizens by right as citizens of former colonies – it is not so now. He started his new life in Reading but could not find any work that made use of his skills. His degrees meant nothing here in the UK. While in Reading, he worked with friends and relatives from Sierra Leone to help incoming refugees and asylum seekers in that area and became very knowledgeable about our immigration laws and procedures, with all their failings. It was then that he met and married Issata Sarah Kallon, a refugee from the north of Sierra Leone. They soon had a daughter, Mariama, who was the apple of his eye.

The family moved to Plymouth for Sam to do more studies in the hope he could get his architecture qualifications recognised. I was introduced to them by a mutual friend who had known them in Reading, and I loved them dearly from the start. They lived in a small council flat in a rough part of Devonport, and were battling valiantly to make a good life for themselves and their daughter, by now four years old. Anyway, I befriended them, and was startled one day when Sam said, 'I hope you don't mind but I have put your name on my papers as next of kin in England; you see, we have no one else.' I was deeply flattered and vowed to be there to support them always. There were many ups and downs but together we pushed ahead and founded (or Sam did) the Devon and Cornwall Refugee Support Council (DCRSC) in Plymouth.

Central government was seeking to disperse asylum seekers to cities other than London, Leeds and Birmingham and they had come up with Plymouth as a good place to send them. Someone thought there must be plenty of

278

empty housing available. So hundreds of weary, dishevelled young men, mostly Kurdish, were sent by bus to Plymouth and accommodated in shabby, crowded housing. Support from the Council was minimal. Who was to educate the children, teach English, help them to find jobs and ensure they received entitled benefits? The answer was us, and we opened our now well-known drop-in help centre, 'The Masiandae Centre,' giving it an African name meaning 'let's help each other'.

DCRSC was born in the Kallon house but soon a group of us helped find premises given generously by the Plymouth Wesley Church, where we stayed for three years, before moving to the present location in central Plymouth. We formed a small group of trustees and started the complicated process of registering as a charity and registering with the Immigration Commissioner as an advice group for asylum seekers.

## Health Unlimited, post- retirement

I had been a trustee of the NGO Health Unlimited (HU) for some years and Chair of their Board for two years. Health Unlimited focused its work on provision of health care to the most remote areas and people most in need, anywhere in the world – always working with local government to build up their capacity to provide long-term care. This work fitted very well with my own principles so I was keen to support them in whatever way I could. Soon after retirement I offered myself as a consultant reviewer if they had need of me.

## China, January 2000

I was asked to take off my trustee's hat and go to China as a volunteer consultant, and was very excited by this prospect. For this, my first assignment for Health Unlimited, I was asked to review a project in a rural district in a remote Burmese border region and to plan with Chinese health officers how to continue the work. It was doubly interesting as the work, supported from China across the Burma border, was undercover and not known about by Burmese authorities.

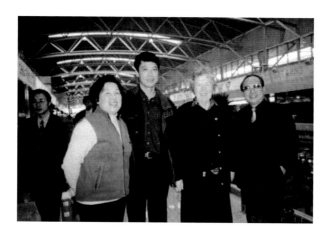

*China – My welcome to Beijing, 2000*

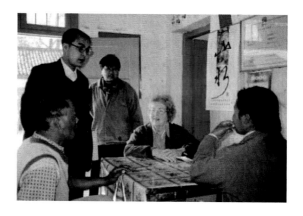

*Talking with a 'barefoot doctor' in China*

The border area was a restricted place for all foreigners and we were surprised and pleased to be given permission to visit; we were watched all the time by what seemed to be a bodyguard of armed soldiers, but when I asked about them, I was always told they were police, and that I must ensure we passed all the checkpoints. They did not intrude – other than when we wanted natural comfort breaks.

280

The aim of the project was to meet the basic, essential health care needs of all women and children living in nine poor, minority counties of Yunnan Province and to prevent epidemic disease in those areas.

An external team of two Health Unlimited technical advisers, Dr Zhu Wei Xing and myself, and two Yunnan provincial technical staff undertook the review. An initial briefing meeting was held with the Province Health Bureau, who had prepared excellent review documentation.

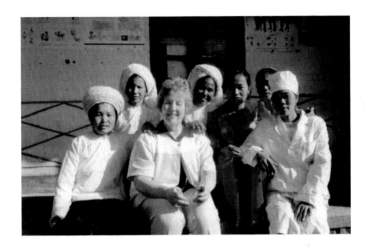

*With village health workers, China*

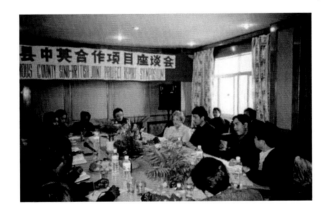

*Conference in China, 2000*

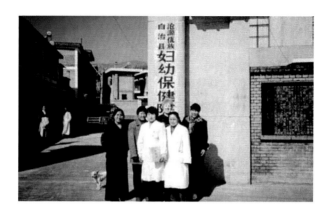

*Field visit, Cangyuan*

Two representative project counties (Shuangbai and Cangyuan) were chosen for field visits – both were 'second phase' counties and they were considered to be representative of conditions and performance in the nine project counties. An internal provincial evaluation had preceded this visit. It was a high quality and detailed assessment of the project work and its results were available to the team. Detailed discussions were held with local government and technical specialists in each county and the team in each place provided feedback at the end of the visit.

A final round-up meeting was held with the Province Health Bureau at the review end. Thus my team was small: just two of us from HU, one of whom was Chinese, and the rest health officials from the Yunnan State Health Department. Working with the latter was very interesting in itself. We had many discussions about healthcare in China and especially what had happened to the famous bare-foot doctor scheme, which had really collapsed. They said it was because they all wanted to be proper doctors and now charged villagers for the care they could give. The only solution suggested was to train women village health volunteers to tackle the vast maternal health problem in the villages.

With help from HU field workers and funds, the project had set up 'Mother and Child Rescue Teams' in all the counties and very good work had been done everywhere. The teams were led from the mother-and-child hospitals (MCH) by obstetric and paediatrics specialists. They were highly dependent on the project vehicles or other available transport; provision of funds for fuel by local government; good communication with township and village health workers; and project equipment for resuscitation and operating.

In both counties, we made visits to village clinics, township hospitals and the county MCH hospital. Village leaders, village women, village doctors (male and female), township doctors and specialist doctors were all interviewed, though time available was short. On my visit I focused my attention very much on women's health matters, and as a team we had many brainstorm sessions on what could be done; there was a healthy amount of lateral thinking.

One day when I was high on a mountain visiting a remote village, the mobile phone of the state medical officer with me rang loudly and he went away to talk. When he came back to me, he exclaimed, 'They can reach you everywhere – even here!' I thought long and hard about that and then put it to the team, that if mobile phones worked out there, then why not just give a phone to every village to call for help when a woman has problems? All right in principle, they thought, but practically, who would go out to help them? The rescue teams could theoretically be used, but they would need more ambulances and emergency-trained doctors and nurses. The result of all this was that we/they set up a trial project of 'flying squads' to rush out in response to calls from villages. There were grave doubts about the terrible roads or tracks and the inaccessibility of villages in this remote mountainous district. I have not heard the outcome of this programme and wish I could go back to find out.

Then we were given a day off. The local officers wanted to show me something interesting. The trouble was it was high on a mountainside and they doubted my ability to walk up there. I had no idea what it was, but decided a day's exploring would be fun. My fellow-women on the team – all Chinese – were apprehensive and did not promise to get all the way. So we drove a long way into the big mountains and stopped at a place where a broad path led upwards. Up we climbed; it was a beautiful, though hard, walk up through tropical forest. After a couple of hours ('just a bit further!'), we came out under a cliff face and I was asked to admire the frescoes. When I had caught my breath, I tried to see them. They were there, but all covered up by trees and bushes growing out of the cliff. It took a lot of looking, but after walking around and looking a bit, what I could see was fascinating.

They were sepia-coloured paintings or line-drawings, clearly old. I asked a lot of questions and wondered whether I was seeing some undiscovered treasure but I was assured that many foreigners had seen them and taken photographs. I did the same and I even researched them when I got home – rather unsuccessfully. I can only compare them to the painting at Les Eyzies in France or some of the aboriginal drawing on the rocks of the Flinders Ranges in South Australia.

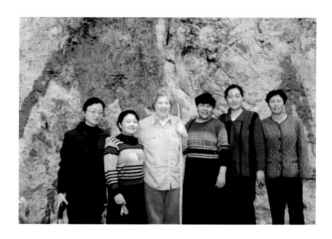

*With Chinese women colleagues up the mountain,*
*in front of the rock drawings*

It started to rain and we slipped our way down, after which the Chinese said they had arranged a Chinese feast for us in a local village and they would be the cooks. I wondered what we were in for. What it turned out to be was a cross between a barbecue and a fondue – or a Cambodian Suki soup. They built a fire and boiled water in a huge iron pot – or trough - over the fire. Then they started putting things in to cook. First meat – mostly goat but some sheep; then vegetables – sweet potatoes, taro and yam; then beans and then green leaves of all sorts; then prawns and fish; what a stew it was! All served up with rice and washed down with local beer. They loved it and I survived it. I hope I showed my pleasure well enough, but I was very tired when we got home very late from our day off.

We visited the district hospital, where every bed was occupied and every patient being given intravenous infusion. When I asked why, there was great surprise and I was told that all patients routinely had intravenous so that medicines could be given correctly. It was expensive, but the patients bought the bottles and the tubes from the pharmacy. Rows of children were being given cocktails of antibiotics for unspecified chest infections. My attempts at suggesting different treatment fell on very deaf ears. They considered me ignorant, I'm sure.

Then we were driven back, with our armed police escort, across the mountains and down the huge Mekong River to the far south of Yunnan almost on the Laos border. I was fascinated to visit a lovely garden full of tropical plants I had seen mainly in Thailand before. The people here were sometimes Khmer speaking, though basically Lao. I understand that Lao people are very close to Khmer. We were driven back to Kunming and had big debriefing sessions with the state health chiefs, who were pretty amazed that we had bothered to go out there or wanted to help those vulnerable people.

In brief, we found that major constraints to project progress were the communications, terrain and distances in the project counties; lack of local government funds for normal recurrent costs such as salaries; lack of village-level health staff, especially women; and lack of community awareness and involvement in their own health care.

We found that community mobilization for health was the weakest area of the project. Also, there was very little contact or communication on a regular basis between the nine project counties. They were missing opportunities to learn from each other.

We were duly fêted at a huge State dinner before reluctantly transferring to the airport for our return home. HU is still working in this part of China.

# Rwanda 2001

Soon after this, I was delighted to be asked to review the Health Unlimited media programme in Rwanda. I had never been there in all my travels, though of course I had followed events there, particularly because of the resemblance to Cambodia.

I visited with the HU regional manager, Jerry, and the local project manager, Josephine. Health Unlimited had developed a successful radio programme in partnership with the BBC in London. It was a 'soap', with story line by a Rwandan writer and local actors to tape the episodes, which were sent back to London for editing before going out on local radio. I was fascinated. I watched the team making the tapes and talked with the writer. I heard that he sought input from local health officers, WHO and UNICEF on programme content.

Then my job was to go out to the villages to find out what impact it was having; who was listening, and had it changed behaviour at all? The story was influenced by local health organisations as well as the health department, who used the programme to publicise subjects like family planning and AIDS.

So our team went off travelling through Rwanda. It is a beautiful country, though scarred forever by the mass graves that were dug hurriedly during and after the civil war of 1994. There was still much fear and distrust of each other, all based on tribal differences and warring, but the villages were largely normal places with the poor farmers going about their work, struggling with drought, as in so much of Africa then.

I remember I was surprised and pleased at the awareness of the people about the radio programme. It was almost famous and had a big following, a bit like *The Archers* in the UK. Well done, the BBC and HU! Health Unlimited went on to replicate this work in Ethiopia and Cambodia, where the audience focus was young people.

At the end of my visit, my task was to go back to Nairobi to the regional office to work with HU staff to develop another project phase to send to potential funders, such as DFID, the EU and even US AID. I am glad to say we were successful and the project continued.


## And Cambodia IV

This land and people have become so much part of my life, and I have been fortunate to maintain close links – and frequent visits. When I left Geneva in early 1999, I went almost directly to Cambodia, where I had been invited to work again for DFID to assist the Ministry of Health to write a new Five-year Health Plan. I was very happy to work on a methodology to do this. Within a week we had agreed a methodology and timeframe. There would be several visits for me and some other consultants over about two years. Our actual start was not to be until 2001.

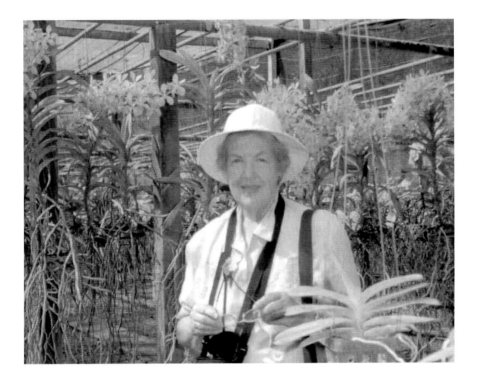

*In Chiang Mai 1998*

## Cambodia new Health Plan 2001-3

It felt quite like old times, but under better and friendlier conditions, to be back with the MOH. A Planning Group or Team had been established as a side-shoot of the original Planning Team I knew so well. I was not so happy with this arrangement as it seemed to me very likely to result in discord (which it did) between the MOH Planning Unit and a new, better paid group of consultants and Cambodians drawn from different departments of MOH,

287

all supposed to be experts in one field or other to render them useful in drawing up a new Five-year Plan.

It took weeks – months – to settle down together as a team. I was fortunate to be working alongside a very experienced British Planning Consultant, Stephanie, whom I had known from my early years with ODA, and in whom I had great confidence to progress our group. She did make the group work hard: no late starts or long lunch breaks for these well-paid experts, whether from Cambodia or overseas! They responded slowly as they understood their roles. We had to undertake a few field trips, mostly to consult with key officials in various departments, like the Ministry of Finance or Education; also Provincial Health Directors, who would be crucial in implementing the Plan we developed. We reported weekly to the Minister, whose baby this was. We set out a 'Road Map' to guide our work and pushed the team hard to meet their/our targets. We were set to produce draft one in six months, but what a lot of work was entailed, and we were back to English/Khmer translation as the Plan had to be produced in Khmer and English.

Stephanie and I both had other jobs to do and so we arranged a series of inputs, tailored to the availability of each of us. After starting up the work I returned again in August 2002, when it was very hot, to review the draft.

During my evenings and weekends I was able to spend time with 'my' family: Kan, Huot and their children. I stayed in their Phnom Penh house mostly when in that city. I enjoyed having a room of my own and a good desk to work at and somewhere to leave my belongings for the next visit. I did not travel to Siem Reap then to see building progress on the house, but just listened to graphic accounts and saw pictures of the construction. I longed to go and see and began to plan my continued involvement in Cambodia, working for or with DFID, the UN, or voluntary organisations, in order to be able to get my air fare paid.

I returned to Cambodia again in early 2002 to help the group and other consultants finalise and review the finished document and then to present it at two big meetings. The whole plan was divided into four volumes, presented in both printed documents (Khmer and English) and on CD.

# West Africa 2002

*This is a personal note about a method that has become important to me in my work over the years.*

Before retiring as DFID health adviser, I had been involved in funding and monitoring various projects being undertaken by the Liverpool School of Tropical Medicine in conjunction with African partners, mostly in the Gambia and Ghana after my retirement from DFID. Paul, the lead researcher, asked me to help him develop a proposal for funding for DFID or others to look at the broad issue of how to translate research findings into revised policies and practices on the ground. For instance, many studies had proved conclusively that measles in young children could be prevented and deaths from measles averted by infant immunisation. But many countries had still not revised their immunisation schedules to include measles injections in early life.

We wanted to know how governments and ministries of health were influenced and changed as a result of new findings. So we planned a visit to several countries to set up a fact-finding project with the aim of supporting country governments to apply new discoveries to their practices.

We visited Senegal, the Gambia, Mali, Ghana and Nigeria and met with senior scientists, researchers and government officials and ministers. At the end of the three months, we developed our partnership of institutions in countries of that region and the subsequent project became GRIPP.

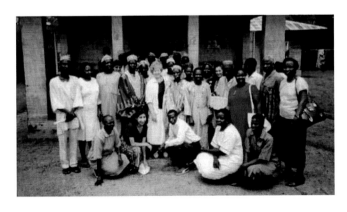

*In rural Africa —at the local government headquarters*

289

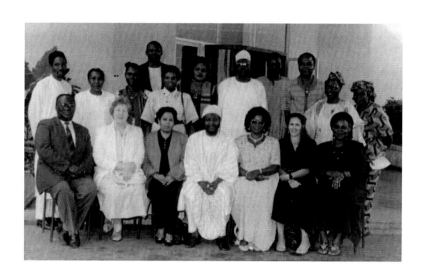

*On a health visit to Nigeria*
*Below – With my two doctor colleagues in Lagos*

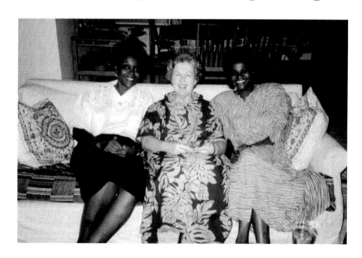

I maintain to this day that without a GRIPP methodology (Getting Research Into Policy And Practice), there is little advantage in medical research. I have yet to find out the results of the study. I had been very privileged to meet so many distinguished and outstanding people, but in all countries my previous work there helped enormously with making contacts and meeting the right people.

# India, June 2003

I was delighted to be asked by DFID to represent them at a special meeting of the Tropical Medical Research Board to be held in Hyderabad, India. I had long experience of this annual meeting and was familiar with the excellent, cutting-edge work being done by the programmes. I was very pleased to return to India, where I knew some of the medical scientists and officials. It was a very pleasant visit, though quite hard work, as I was elected rapporteur for the meeting.

# Cambodia 2003

In late 2003, during one of my health plan visits, I was approached by Health Unlimited to help them to develop and write a new project they had been invited to bid for by MOH. It was for management and technical support of a project to develop the provincial health services – funded by the World Bank. Already MOH had piloted this approach in two provinces with some success. Now they wanted to extend the approach to remote and poorly served provinces – Ratanakiri, Mmondulkiri, Preah Vihear and Koh Kong. HU wished to bid for Ratanakiri and I was to carry out preparatory work and write the bid. I agreed to return in April/May to complete the work, but was suddenly asked by another NGO, Healthnet International (HNI), to come to their rescue at once to complete their bid for the work in Ratanakiri. Here was a dilemma and potential inter-agency conflict. I discussed with both agencies, with the result that the bid for Ratanakiri work would include a partnership of the two of them, sharing out the areas of strength of each. But the deadline for submission was very close when I started and I had limited time for all the groundwork needed, so I went ahead with both, using a small team of Cambodian staff to gather statistics that I needed and to help with methodology ideas. I had to go home a week before the deadline and remember writing as I travelled home on the plane and finalising the bid at home, sending lots of zipped files as there was no broadband then. I was pleased that HNI won their bid and HU won theirs for Preah Vihear. I have heard that both projects went well. This had taken me a total of three months work and I was quite tired, but there was more to come…

# National AIDS Authority, Cambodia.

In 2004, I was asked by DFID Cambodia to help sort out a systems problem within the new agency established in Phnom Penh to cope with all services for HIV/AIDS and known as the National AIDS Authority. It had been set up as a political response to the growing crisis and had been made directly responsible to the Council of Ministers, outside the MOH. This had proved very unwise as it was no one's job to monitor and supervise its work. No one had ever decided what role it was to play, and in particular what were its relations with the MOH programmes already under implementation. DFID was a major donor to the AIDS programme there and had agreed with other main donors (USAID and Germany) that plans had to be formed and institutional systems established.

Looking back, I think it was one of the most difficult of my assignments in Cambodia. The Director was an inspirational leader but could not manage an institution and the staff thought I was out to cut their jobs and salaries and did not want to cooperate with me. I really struggled. It took me two long assignments over 18 months to come to an agreed structure and a Plan of Action. Looking back, I believe this was one of the several stress periods leading up to my stroke.

# Stover

And so to write of Stover School, which my mother founded and which I attended between the ages of thirteen and seventeen years. For many years I have been a governor (and trustee), as when I returned to work in London for ODA, I was asked to become a governor in place of my mother who had just retired. I was not able to attend regularly because of being out of the country so much, but my fellow governors were good enough to give me leave of absence and allow me to remain on the board. Indeed, this was one of the reasons why I had picked on Bovey Tracey to retire to. I wanted to be near Stover so that I could be a better governor and attend school events and meetings more frequently. So this I now did in earnest.

I was genuinely very interested and enjoy the company of young people and staff. I was Chair of Governors for three years, during which time I had my stroke. We had had a very difficult year, as there were a lot of problems to solve and I think that this, too, did actually add to the stress which led to my stroke. Now things are much better and again, I really enjoy the life of the school. I have felt a part of the Stover community, which has always been very rewarding. I still continue as a governor, although I think I am probably now too old to make a huge contribution. But I am assured by my fellow governors that I can still be of use – my long experience counts for something.

## Malaria Consortium, London

Over these years, my interests in overseas health matters have continued, and one of them led to a very rewarding involvement. My good friend and malaria expert, Sylvia, came to me one day asking for my help in the dire situation she found herself and her malaria project in. She had been working at the London School of Hygiene and Tropical Medicine to support an area programme in West Africa being funded by a grant from ODA (now DFID). The funding had been stopped, quite suddenly, and she was very upset, not so much for herself, but for the work being done that would have to stop without the funding. She saw a real need for another non-governmental organisation based in the UK, providing support to the many countries where the burden of malaria is still extreme. After a lot of discussion, both with her and with other people, I agreed to help her to set up a new malaria charitable organisation. I felt I had some experience in a venture like this in my work in Plymouth.

The first job was to find a group of people to become trustees to the organisation to manage and govern it. Only then could we set about applying for funding grants so that we could employ some staff. Sylvia and I both worked hard to find a suitable group of like-minded people. Actually, we achieved this and brought onto the board some extremely knowledgeable people who had the same concern as we did for the malaria burden in the world. Two of my ex-ODA colleagues came to help, and they have both been extraordinarily useful in establishing the organisation and improving relations with government organisations like DFID.

We achieved a lot and in 2002 the **Malaria Consortium** was borne. The next important task was to find a chairman or woman with a high profile and good connections. Most of the professors and deans of colleges and universities who would meet these requirements were far too busy, even if they were willing, to take on this role for this risky new organisation. My mind turned to a paediatrician I had worked with on the India programme. He had now been elevated to the peerage, and so I approached Lord Michael Chan to help us. Lord Chan's life and work had been dedicated to improving the health and lifestyle of the poorest people. He had particular knowledge and interest in Asia (from where he came), and where the burden of communicable diseases, including malaria, is very high. Quickly, he took over as chairman (a role I had been fulfilling as an interim) and made a huge difference to the early years of the organisation. Sadly, he died quite suddenly, after only two years with us. But by this time the organisation had taken off well. Malaria Consortium offices had been established in East Africa and Ghana.

Now I am a proud trustee, working with a new, dynamic chairman, MP Stephen O'Brien, who has helped enormously to develop our communication with Parliament and with world leaders. He has an exciting vision for Malaria Consortium, which is ever changing to do more in the world. I am proud of it and hope to continue with it for a while.

## My Stroke

As has been indicated, I had a stroke, and for one year of convalescence I could not think more than about regaining my independence, but I still had to try a visit (of course!) to Cambodia. My adopted family were missing me and my advice in their venture; the children growing up, getting married, graduating, falling in love and giving their parents anxious moments. So I determined to travel and could only manage when my dear friend Brenda said she would go with me as she planned a visit too. So in August 2005 I had a big adventure, flying again – with good wheelchair assistance all the way. I loved being back but did find it all a struggle. I was not very mobile and I had several bad falls. It was lovely being with the family again and, though glad to return home, I would not have missed it.

Then I took a big decision to sell *Hestia*. I had resisted this immediately after my stroke, mostly because my friends and relatives all said, 'Don't make any rush decision – wait and consider.' Now was the time to make that decision. I was getting more mobile and very restless to have the house to myself again (which I could not do with an upstairs bedroom), and to get into my garden, but it was on the side of a steep hill and I just couldn't manage. I was still falling a good deal; falling hurt and I could not get up by myself. I considered all the pros and cons and discussed them with helpful friends, who understood.

In spring 2007 I put my house up for sale. I was just in time, before the dreadful slump. As I needed to buy again I had to get a good price, even though I would downsize. I needed a ground floor apartment with good access and a bit of garden and I really wanted to stay in Bovey Tracey. There was nothing in sight even when my sale went through at the end of the year. Then I found one: a really nice, spacious flat on the ground floor of a big house, converted into six flats; more than that, it had its own garden. I knew it was for me when I first went in. I just needed to get a price reduction as the bathroom needed adapting for me. But by God's grace, it all went through and I moved in just two weeks after leaving *Hestia*. Even the adaptations were finished in time. Packing and unpacking were a nightmare. I survived through the generous help of cousins and friends who came and stayed for a few days in the chaos and sorted thoroughly. It was eight months before my garage was cleared and I could put my car away.

I am happy and independent in my flat and I can manage it, with caring help on a daily basis.

## National Stroke Association

I often read a journal sent me by this organisation. I noticed that they were appealing for lay members for their research awards committee which takes decisions on which research proposals to fund. I was interested as I wanted to do something for other stroke survivors. I went through an interview process and was accepted, despite being a bit dubious about my status as a doctor; but it proved all right and I became a lay member, representing stroke survivors. I get many piles of proposals to read through and comment on – quite like old times! I have to collate the views of several other lay members and present our joint views to the main committee in London, so I attend three meetings a year there. I enjoy these meetings, and find it all very interesting, meeting many experienced stroke experts and scientists and hearing all the latest developments.

## Peninsula Stroke Research Committee.

This is a more local initiative to support stroke specialists in the south-west peninsula. I have only recently started this. It could become very time-consuming.

In addition I have continued as trustee of the Devon and Cornwall Refugee Support Council – also time-consuming, but very interesting. It is close to my heart. I am also still a trustee of the Malaria Consortium with London meetings and a trustee/governor of Stover, so I occupy myself fully and appreciate being wanted still.

This year, 2009, in Cambodia again, I was offered a job. It gave me a huge boost that someone thought I was still capable of work. But it was impractical and I knew I could not cope with the remote travel needed, so I said no.

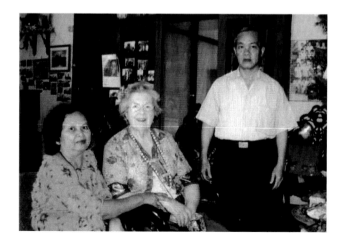

*With Kan and Huot, 2009*

296

# Chapter 13: Reflections

## Being single

My sister Kan asked me recently, 'Who was your man? Why did you not marry?' It set me thinking; but I could honestly say, 'Because the right man did not come along.' In most places I worked overseas it is almost unthinkable for a woman not to be married and, like single friends, I have sometimes replied to the inevitable question and wonder with, 'My husband is in heaven.' That is well understood. If one admits to being single by choice, it is seen as a gross fault by your father, whose duty it is to find you a husband and arrange your future security, since the perception is that marriage is for security and so that you will be looked after.

I once had a proposal from an African chief in Transkei. He did me great honour at that time of apartheid, when he would have been in dreadful trouble from the white South African authorities, jailed at least. I was rather frightened at the time as he was a very powerful man and I thought perhaps he could summon his tribe and force me to the ceremony; but he gave in with dignity and disappeared back to his bunch of wives – some five or six, along with many children.

Earlier I had my flutters like most young women, but my standards were too high. I had a very particular test for sharing my life and broke off with at least one serious contender because of this. It concerned my duty and calling as a doctor. I used to make very clear that any serious relationship would be based on my continuing medical work, as I could not give up my work or stop being 'on call' for a reason such as getting married. Yes, I met some wonderful men whom I respected a lot, but there was always the work issue around, so I made my choice and regretted it at some lonely times, but on the whole, looking back, it was right for me. I describe myself as a professional workaholic career-woman, which does not go well with marriage and motherhood. Something would have had to go. I am a Christian and believe that my choices were God's will and right in His eyes.

297

He will judge me in my next life, when I believe I will meet up with all those I love.

## My Children

To return to my single state; above all I had wanted children and recall vividly a day on holiday in Australia when I knew finally and accepted that I would not have a child of my own. I vowed to make it my mission to 'adopt' or look after vulnerable babies and children and always to keep children in my life. This I have done, by God's grace. I believe it is vitally important for older people, especially if they are on their own, to have a child in their life as an absorbing interest and to keep them young at heart.

## A snapshot of 'my' children:

my nephews and nieces: Ben, Jane and Tom; David and Andrew; Adam, Sophy and Helen; all children of my three brothers, who were generous in that they let me share their children, which meant such a lot to me and still does. To them I have dedicated this work, and I treasure many faded photos of them, some with torn or curled edges, as they were pinned on walls wherever I happened to be. Now there are also their children, my great-nephews and great-nieces, including Clare and Laura, the latest but possibly not last additions;

my dear godchildren: Ben, David, Helen, Alison, Chris, Clare and Stephen;

and my other 'adopted' children: little Penny in Papua – an abandoned babe I cared for for two years. She was profoundly deaf but otherwise a lovely and playful girl. I could not locate her when I last returned to Dogura. I believe that a local family was found for her; Alison Penelope and Rachel, twin daughters whom I delivered of my best friend, Jean, at Dogura. I so loved these little girls, along with their brother Philip, and sister Jo, who I keep up with now; my namesake in Papua – Penny Sinapa from Wanigela, Lancelot's daughter; my Cambodian orphans: baby Carl, Becca and many more; John Kanya and Kannary, children of my adopted sister, Kan; and Kanrattana Tim, her little boy, and now early in 2009, John's son Davin, and Kannary's little son, Kanjanaran; and last but not least, my dear adopted granddaughter, Mariama.

298

## My protégés from overseas:

Kem Kanyaket, my sister and her husband Huot;

Phalyka Oum – a doctor, and Sophea Oum, her sister, married to an Englishman;

Lina Norng, my long-term helper and friend, and Utara (Tola) Norng, her sister, who came to England to school for a year and who now works for the UN War Crimes Commission in Cambodia.

These are mostly Cambodian, who I still try to support. I love them all and wish them happy and successful lives.


## My African family of orphans:

Hassan Joseph, Steven, Mamadu Andrew, Neneh Theresa, Isatta Penny, and Abu Peter.

These are the children of Issatta Sarah's sister, also from Sierra Leone. We found them, after a long search, in a refugee camp in Ghana. Just after we found them, Sarah's sister tragically died of malaria in Ghana, so the small children were left motherless. After a lot of negotiation with the British Embassy in Ghana, I managed to get them visas to come to the UK under the Family Reunion scheme. Sarah went out to meet them and I met them at Gatwick Airport. They are now settled in this country.


## Called to serve and always make a difference

When I took up my desk job in London, and for the next twenty years, I accepted that my direct 'saving lives' days were over. I had been there and done that. Now I had to find other better ways to make a difference. A high proportion of my work was about training people or training people to train people. I found ways to support and develop training schools: nursing schools, medical schools and post graduate training. I worked alongside British hospital and medical school consultants to advise and fund the poorest, least-developed countries' health workforces. Ghana, India and the West Indies are good examples; as has been Cambodia recently. I like to think there are quite a few doctors, nurses, lab. technicians and medical consultants who, without my input, would not now be able to make a difference to their own countries and people.

As well, I found myself working to develop the next generation of health advisers to help our UK government spend their development money wisely and on health services development and workforces. It pleases me greatly that the current health advisers were recruited in my time and are where they are because of my encouragement. Many of my protégés and colleagues have senior posts in the UN, notably in WHO, where they will now be hugely influential professionals; thus I have made a difference once removed.

Close to home, within my immediate family, I undoubtedly influenced my brother John to venture out into the third world. He has helped so many people in different ways to me so it must have mattered. His son Ben, who is in the Royal Navy, clearly has a heart to help people develop their skills, wherever they may come from. He has time yet to get into developing defence systems in other countries. My brother Tim had his own life and career at home in Devon. I sometimes feel guilty (though proud) that his two sons have both travelled the world and worked in various developmental areas. David cleared mines in Angola and Afghanistan, not the most comfortable countries for anxious parents or aunts, and Andrew, after visiting me in Cambodia in his GAP year, entered the Foreign and Commonwealth Office and has risen fast, after a long posting in China. My MP brother Rob was Parliamentary Private Secretary to Chris Patten, Minister of Overseas Development. I had the pleasure of watching him get to understand a bit what development is about and why I had been committed to it all my career. Then his son Adam, who had also spent several months with me in Cambodia, started to roam the world in the course of his financial career. I have yet to hear that he is tackling the finance systems of developing countries; but it is very much needed. The children of the next generation are growing up, but are all too young to think about careers. It is the fashion to go and see the world, but I say to them and many young people, wait until you have a skill to pass on and then think where and how you can make a difference to people who do not have your privileges.

Who knows, perhaps one day far in the future, just one more Key family girl or woman may follow in my footsteps to carry on the task of improving the well-being of women and children in far-off places. If this account of my life encourages such a decision, then it too will have made a difference.


## My Faith/My Vine

When I was thirteen years old, my aunt, Phyllis Dence, gave me some verses of scripture to guide my life. They were from St John's gospel:

*'I am the true vine, and my Father is the gardener. He cuts off every branch in me that bears no fruit, while every branch that does bear fruit he prunes so that it will be even more fruitful; you are already clean because of the word I have spoken to you. Remain in me, and I will remain in you. No branch can bear fruit by itself; it must remain in the vine. Neither can you bear fruit unless you remain in me. I am the vine; you are the branches. If a man (or woman) remains in me and I in him, he will bear much fruit; apart from me you can do nothing. If anyone does not remain in me, he is like a branch that is thrown away and withers; such branches are picked up, thrown into the fire and burned. If you remain in me and my words remain in you, ask whatever you wish, and it will be given you. This is to my Father's glory, that you bear much fruit, showing yourselves to be my disciples.*

*As the Father has loved me, so have I loved you. Now remain in my love. If you obey my commands, you will remain in my love, just as I have obeyed my Father's commands and remain in his love. I have told you this so that my joy may be in you and that your joy may be complete. My command is this: Love each other as I have loved you. Greater love has no-one than this, that he lay down his life for his friends. You are my friends if you do what I command. I no longer call you servants, because a servant does not know his master's business. Instead, I have called you friends, for everything that I learned from my Father I have made known to you. You did not choose me, but I chose you and appointed you to go and bear fruit that will last. Then the Father will give you whatever you ask in my name. This is my command: Love each other.'*

St John Chapter 15 v 1-17

At first I thought little of these, but as my career and faith developed I kept going back to the verses and they did become my guide and delight in all my jobs, wherever I was until now and beyond. Looking back, I see:

## Branches cut off because no fruit

*'He cuts off every branch in me that bears no fruit.'* On reflection this is when I stopped clinical practice to move into public health. I did not want to at the time but was led to make the transition, so I believe that God had a role in this and a purpose. Perhaps I had come to the limit of what I could do in that field? And was not doing very good work? I know I was burnt out with excess clinical workload, especially in Africa, my last clinical posting. I don't see it as wasted vine. There was strong growth and fruit at the time but God pruned that branch for a purpose, that I should be of more use in another branch of medicine where I could make a bigger difference in His purpose.

The other branch that was pruned and not allowed to grow was family – having a husband and children of my own. If He had designed this for me, then it would have happened one way or another, but that fruit was not to be mine and instead I gained much and I did much for other vulnerable families and children. In the end it was my gain and I hope theirs.

## Pruning

Early work years. After five or six years of hard slogging at medical school, followed by resident hospital jobs in general medicine, surgery, obstetrics and gynaecology, it would have been reasonable to settle down into a steady medical job at home, using what I had learned. Instead I plunged into what proved to be a huge experience of learning new skills. A lot of the old skills fell away early; I suppose they were cut off to make room for the new?

302

# My growing vine

This was characterized by my world journeys and my medical work – wherever I made a difference to other people – represented here by my condensed curriculum vitae.

- My early experience included fifteen years' hands-on clinical work in the third world (Papua New Guinea; Cambodia; Transkei), district-level health care, specialising in tropical diseases and women and children's health care.
- I was awarded Order of the British Empire in 1977 for services to Cambodian children. I regarded this as an award for my whole team, not only me.
- In the 1980s, I became involved in the broader international health development scene; employed for twenty years in HM Civil Service in various technical posts and locations, including India and Cambodia, from a base at the Department for International Development (then the ODA) in London.
- During the 1980s-90s, I developed expertise in communicable disease control, reproductive health and the development and management of health systems in Asia, Africa (Nigeria, Ghana, Angola, Sierra Leone) and the Pacific, especially in post-conflict and resource-starved countries.
- I developed special interest in health sector institutional development and human resource capacity strengthening, especially in post-conflict situations; this has developed a wide network of institutional and professional contacts in Britain and internationally.
- I gained experience in both government and non-government settings overseas; interactive at top-level with governments, health ministries and international organisations (WHO; UNDP; UNICEF).
- I engaged in strategic initiatives on behalf of global and regional development agencies, including WHO in Geneva and the Balkans and UN in Cambodia, St Helena and West Africa.

- I was appointed Trustee for four International Health Development Agencies: Malaria Consortium (current); Health Unlimited; Healthlink Worldwide; MERLIN. I was also Health Adviser to: the USPG; Diana, Princess of Wales, Memorial Fund; Comic Relief; and the Nuffield Foundation. I was elected Chair of Trustees of the Devon & Cornwall Refugee Support Council.

## My withering vine

*'apart from me you can do nothing. If anyone does not remain in me, he is like a branch that is thrown away and withers; such branches are picked up, thrown into the fire and burned'.*

I feel now that my work in Transkei and Zaire led to little. I hear disturbing news of happenings in Transkei and the health services there. I don't think I made much difference in the long term. Zaire was probably a mistake for me as it was not development work, just reactive clinical care. I went there for the wrong reason – to earn money, rather than to serve. I think there was nothing left behind other than a few mother and child lives saved; for individuals a lot; but for the country as a whole, little.

Is it finished? I don't think so. I am waiting to hear what is next. *'You did not choose me, but I chose you and appointed you to go and bear fruit that will last.'*

I ask myself now: will it all last? Will my vine still bear fruit and spread, or is it time it was cut down and allowed to wither and die? I don't think so. Rather, I have positive thoughts about my new life. I suffered my stroke three years ago. Now, this far on, I live alone as before – with limitations. I've learned that I must come to terms with the difference. At times now I feel really well just like before, only my left hand has yet to respond well – but it will, of this I am sure. God will heal me in His time – not mine. I just keep trying and use all the wonderful help I have. People here have been so good to me. I have reviewed my last two Independent Living Plans and can report joyfully that I have achieved most of what I set myself. I count my blessings often.

304

It is a good new life! I still so badly want to be useful to someone. I am not going to sit at home. I always intended to keep up my interests and travel in my retirement. This is not the time to stop.

My motto is, 'I can do it with God's help'. People everywhere help me as I go out and about and I let them and welcome help.

Don't anyone be surprised at what I will do next. I am not one to sit around and be sorry for myself. My lifework has been serving others less fortunate than myself and there are still plenty of them out there.

In ten years' time when I am past eighty years, perhaps I will have another book to write? Only God knows and I know that the young of my extended family are already carrying on the tradition established many years ago by Keys and Dences and will fulfil an old family motto (courtesy of the Beale family):

'People will not look forward to posterity
Who never look backwards to their ancestors'

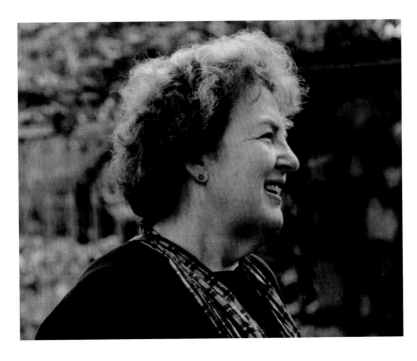

*Looking forward*

# Appendix 1

## Cambodian health in transition

Mam Bun Heng, P J Key

As conflict and suffering in Bosnia, Chechnya, Rwanda, and Zaire continue to be at the forefront of world attention, some countries seem to be largely forgotten. It is timely to take stock of conditions in the small country of Cambodia as it struggles to take its place after a long period of isolation. Countless Cambodians and ethnic Vietnamese have died there this year and during the past 25 years, victims of senseless killing or preventable disease.

Early in 1975 one of us (PJK) led a relief team of 200 health workers, 190 of them Cambodians, taking medical care and food supplements to a million or so women and children who were refugees in besieged Phnom Penh. Later that year all expatriates were evicted from the country by the advancing forces of Pol Pot. On re-establishing contact in 1980 we found that only 12 of the original Cambodian team had survived. Their stories of suffering and killing, and of escape and survival, under the murderous regime that followed are harrowing. Cambodia now has a fast growing population of around 9 million, a fifth of whom are children under 5 years old. Their health and safety are still precarious.

### Background

The past 20 years of Cambodian history have been characterised by civil war and terrible brutality. In the early 1970s the country suffered intense bombing by the United States on its western border with Vietnam. The fall of Phnom Penh to the Khmer Rouge marked the beginning of four years of genocide under the rule of Pol Pot; the country was turned into a "killing field", with up to two million people dying as the result of violence, starvation, and disease. In 1979 the Vietnamese ended Pol Pot's rule and installed a hardline socialist regime. Over the next 10 years Cambodia suffered a vicious civil war as the government in Phnom Penh battled with guerrilla factions backed by the West. The long period of civil disturbance and conflict left many more thousands dead or disabled.

The public health infrastructure was another casualty of these decades of violence. Under Pol Pot the Cambodian professional classes were destroyed to the extent that only 25 doctors and three members of staff at the ministry of health remained. Although the new regime backed by the Vietnamese tried to train large numbers of health workers quickly, the training was not accredited to international standards and its quality was untested and questionable. Other distortions also emerged. Salaries for all government staff were below a living wage, with doctors earning about $US30 a month in 1992. Low incomes had to be supplemented by private practice, which was most lucrative in towns. Few doctors were prepared to work in rural areas, where health problems were gravest and purchasing power the lowest.

Thus a two tier health service has emerged. On the one hand, is the public sector, which is badly underfunded. Health facilities are in disrepair and without water, electricity, equipment, or drugs; staff are present for only a few hours each day and always try to make patients pay a fee. Thus only a few patients are treated. On the other hand, there is the private sector, which is thriving in the towns (usually in private houses), with quality and cost totally unregulated.

**Health indicators**

Cambodia has some of the worst health indicators in Asia. Although no firm data are available, the ministry of health estimates that life expectancy is about 47 years for men and 49 years for women, infant mortality 120 per 1,000 live births, child mortality 190 per 1,000, and maternal mortality nine per 1,000 births. Because many men were killed in the conflicts, there are more women than men of reproductive age, and over a fifth of households are headed by a woman.

Many of the diseases that kill Cambodians are not new to developing countries. In infants and children these are tetanus, diarrhoeal diseases, acute respiratory infections, haemorrhagic dengue, and diseases that can be prevented by vaccination. Women of reproductive age have complications of pregnancy, abortion and delivery, often superimposed on severe anaemia, undernutrition and malaria. What makes Cambodia different is the scale and complexity of these diseases. For instance, diarrhoea is also a major cause of serious illness in adults, and typhoid and cholera are endemic because access to clean drinking water and latrines is extremely limited everywhere (even in the capital). Then there are the major killers: malaria and tuberculosis.

Cambodian malaria is among the most intransigent and deadly in the world. Malaria (primarily *Plasmodium fakiparuni*) is the single greatest cause of illness and death, with an estimated half a million cases each year and between 5,000 and 10,000 deaths. About a fifth of maternal deaths are attributed to malaria. The ministry of health estimates that up to a third of all Cambodians are at serious risk of malaria. The remote forested areas, where health services are weakest and security is poorest, are the worst affected. Recent mass movements of people, poor compliance with drug regimens and unregulated dispensing of antimalarial drugs in the private sector have contributed to drug resistance that is regarded by the World Health Organisation as among the most serious in the world.

The annual incidence of pulmonary tuberculosis is estimated to be 250 per 100,000 people. This means that every year 40,000 new cases are expected, of which 20,000 will have sputum that is positive for *Mycobacterium tuberculosis*. Of these 40,000 new cases each year, an estimated 11,000 will be treated but only 4,400 of affected patients will complete the full course. Shortage of drugs, failure to complete the course of treatment, inadequacy of the 12 month protocol, and growing drug resistance limit the effectiveness of the national tuberculosis control programme.

The rapid spread of HIV infection in South East Asia poses a formidable challenge to Cambodia. Neighbouring Thailand has one of the highest infection rates in the world, and the prevalence is increasing in Vietnam. Cambodia is likewise showing all the signs of an exponential rise in HIV infection rates. Recent sample surveys show that the prevalence of HIV infection is over 50% in commercial sex workers in some areas, and about 10% in the police and armed forces. Blood donors testing HIV positive have increased from under 1% in the early 1990s to 4% in 1994. The presence of a large United Nations peace keeping force from early 1992 to the end of 1993 and the easing of the political and economic situation have brought in their wake a fast growing commercial sex industry. The large shifts in population for political and economic reasons, returning refugees, and the porous borders with neighbouring countries have also bolstered HIV transmission.

The history of violence has left a legacy unique to Cambodia: large numbers of disabled people and about 13 million land mines in a land of 9 million people. There are about 20,000 people with amputations in the country; each month between 100 and 200 people have a limb amputated and a further 200 or so die of injuries caused by land mines. Local manufacturing capacity for prostheses is limited, and in any case artificial limbs are a valuable resaleable commodity among the poor. As with HIV infection, the young adult population working in fields or forests is at greatest risk of injury.

The Cambodian ministry of health recognises and is much concerned that highly traumatising events such as the prolonged war, the dislocation of families and loss of relatives, and the constant fear of injury from mines have resulted in considerable psychiatric morbidity, with many people in need of psychiatric and counselling services. Studies among displaced Cambodians in border camps show an unusually high incidence of mental ill health. Overstretched resources and limited qualified staff mean, however, that mental health care services are not currently provided and that psychiatry and psychology are not part of the current educational curriculum for health professionals.

## The future

The violence continues. But the Cambodians are trying to re-establish the public health care services, which were almost totally dismantled. This is a priority for national leaders. The signing of the Paris Peace Accord in 1991 ended political isolation and allowed international donors to expand humanitarian initiatives. With the combined efforts of the national government and national and international organisations, particularly non-governmental organisations, parts of the health service have been revitalised rapidly and the transitional phase leading to long term development has begun.

The new royal Cambodian government, with much help from WHO technical experts, has taken important steps to re-establish a viable health care system. With its decimated health care workforce, low level of recurrent finance for health care, and limited managerial capacity, Cambodia has moved rapidly to establish sensible health policies and plans, mechanisms to coordinate external donors, and options to increase the finance available for health care and to improve the use of existing non-governmental health practitioners. The Cambodian ministry of health is one of the first in the world to lead the way for more widespread civil service reform, starting with changes in budget and accounting practice and moving into human resource planning and management. Senior health managers, working closely with the WHO and Unicef, have already earned the respect of professionals in the World Bank, Asian Development Bank, United Nations Development Programme, and major bilateral agencies, all of which are optimistic that Cambodia is pulling through and that there is a reasonable prospect within the next 10 years of establishing an appropriate and sustainable health system, suited to and meeting the needs of the Cambodian people.

There is, however, much more to be done before even a minimum package of primary health care activities is available to all Cambodians. Health services need to aim for reduced financial and technical dependence on external donors and for long term sustainability. This means devising alternative, indigenous methods of financing health services. Although foreign technical skills are available in abundance in Cambodia, what Cambodian health professionals need most now is to see for themselves how other countries in the region have tackled similar problems, and to learn from their experiences. The goals of Cambodia's national health development plan for 1994-6 are, by its own admission, ambitious, but they need to be because "the health needs of [the Cambodian] people are so great."

*Reprinted from the* **BMJ,** *12th August 1995 , Vol. 311, Pages 435-437*
*BMJI252I95* COPYRIGHT © 1995    All rights of reproduction of this reprint are reserved in all countries of the world

# Appendix 2

## Roll-Back Malaria 1998

Outline of the project

The WHO RBM project will contribute to country partnerships by offering help in several areas, including:

i.   possible agreements and means of working;
ii.  materials for advocacy;
iii. help with developing a consensus on strategy – ensuring that options considered are based on best available evidence;
iv.  capacity building;
v.   lesson learning from other countries and from other programmes;
vi.  support for monitoring progress, and
vii. brokering resources (looking for new channels as well as existing ones).

## The Malaria Burden: problems and issues

Malaria affects 100 countries world wide, causing 300-500 million clinical cases per year, over 80% of which are in Africa, and one million deaths per year, over 95% of which are in children under five years in Africa. Severe forms of the disease result in neurological sequelae and disability, the extent of which is probably underestimated but which no doubt has a significant impact on cognitive learning especially among children. The malaria situation is worsening. Malaria has been reintroduced to areas where eradication was achieved in the 1950s and 60s; it is now found in areas previously free of the disease; and the number of epidemics in Africa, Southeast Asia and South America is increasing.

Perhaps the major threat to the control of malaria is the development of drug resistance: to sulphadoxine-primethamine and mefloquine in South East Asia; to chloroquine and, more recently, to sulphadoxine-pyrimethamine in Africa. Other major problems in the control of malaria are poor access to health care and issues associated with delivery, including: under-utilisation of public health facilities and high use of the formal and non-formal private sector; poor availability of antimalarials in public health facilities and high costs.

The basic concept of RBM is to address a priority problem within the context of health sector development, intersectoral collaboration and community action. WHO will provide strategic direction to a global partnership to make the best use of available resources through the RBM project.

## Objectives of the RBM partnership are:

to significantly reduce the global malaria burden through improving people's access to interventions adapted to local needs;

to achieve results through effective support to health sector development;

national goals to be set by countries based on situation analysis and feasibility assessment;

global targets will be set from aggregated national goals at the end of the RBM preparatory phase (end 1999).

## Analysis of global and regional Partnerships for Health
### Dr Penelope Key (January 1999)

An analysis of existing global and regional partnerships which have had varying degrees of success was undertaken in order to identify key characteristics of successful programmes of relevance to establishing the RBM partnership mechanism. Some of these have a public health mandate (polio eradication, UNAIDS) while others address other sectors such as agriculture or the environment. There is a wide spectrum of existing partnership structures and governance, ranging from the tightly governed, legally binding group at one end to the loose stakeholder coalitions at the other end. In the middle sit a large group with a degree of governance and structure, but having a flexible operating modality. The degree of ownership by, or involvement of, countries as equal partners varies from virtual exclusion to full, such as the Intergovernmental Forum on Chemical Safety.

313

Partnerships whose prime purpose or mandate is for raising and managing financial resources, usually centrally operated, tend to be tightly governed, with strict membership rules, legal agreements, management staff and tight criteria for allocation of funds. Partnerships whose primary mandate is co-ordination of strategies and activities, with action taking place at country level, tend (though not always) to be looser, informal coalitions of stakeholders, where secretariat functions are undertaken by programme staff. Partnerships with secretariats that are autonomous or independent of programme management tend to demonstrate better ownership by the partners, but they have sustainability problems.

Where resource mobilisation and management functions are integral to programmes, as in WHO TDR and HRP and WHO GPVI, this has a real cost in terms of staff time and detracts from programme achievements. It appears that there is value in out-placing this function to an independent Partnership Structure. Resource mobilisation must be planned and continuous. Involvement of private (commercial) sector agencies as full members of partnerships may dictate the partnership structure. WHO, for instance, has regulations which exclude their full (voting) membership of certain official committees.

A high-profile Civil Society Champion is invaluable for continued advocacy and resource mobilisation. The roles of each Partner organisation should be defined clearly from the start. Building the partnerships requires time and effort. Continued, consistent information and updating of partners about programme progress is essential. Personal rapport is needed between partners at a high level. Political commitment in endemic countries must be maintained. Inter-sectoral support in countries is vital to public health programmes and requires involvement of the Head of State to succeed.

Regional Partnerships have shown considerable success. The West Africa OCP is the outstanding example. This is firmly sited in the tight governance group. One longstanding collaboration in Asia (SEMEO-TROPMED) is institution-based but has proved its worth, the second (ACTMalaria) has started well but long-term funding is a problem. Regional partnerships will be challenged by agencies' differing regional definitions. In the case of malaria, boundaries based on epidemiological types are more logical. Cross-regional representation is invaluable.

Proposals are made for possible structure of the RBM partnerships based on past experiences and lessons learned.

# Appendix 3

Extract from Pene's thesis:

## THE HEALTH OF ORISSA'S WOMEN
A Review of their Health and Family Welfare.
by Penelope J Key, OBE, MBBS, DTM&H, DRCOG

Department of Tropical Hygiene
University of London

September 1986

## SUMMARY

Orissa is one of the least developed of India's States, with most of its people living in poverty. The women are further disadvantaged by their low status in society, this having special implications for their health. In 1980, a health sector Area Development Programme (ADP) was started in 5 districts of the State and in 1982 a Baseline Household Survey was undertaken covering 1000 households in each district. The Baseline Survey provides information on the health and family welfare status of Orissa's women as well as the extent that needs are being met and makes suggestions for improvements in service delivery.

Orissan women suffer a high level of morbidity and mortality due to frequent, too close and too many pregnancies. Childbirth almost always takes place in the home without skilled attention and complications often occur. General health is threatened by insufficient food intake. Child loss is also high, mostly from malnutrition, diarrhoea and other preventable infections.

The health and family welfare services provided, both by the regular government system and by the ADP, have taken basic health care within reach of the majority of people in the 5 selected districts, which represent almost half the State's population. In these districts family welfare performance has shown improvement over the first years of the programme, but emphasis has been on family planning and on female sterilisation rather than birth spacing, with consequent lower performance in maternal and child care.

Orissan women use health services less than men, even when they are readily accessible; not because their need is less, but because they either do not recognise their need or there are social and economic barriers preventing them. There is a need for better communication in health matters with women in their homes. Trained *dais*, community health volunteers and multi-purpose health workers are seen as having key roles in meeting this need and in promoting women's and children's health.

Although Government has not yet reached a decision on future programmes, it remains important to carry out a further survey to measure this ADP's impact and changes occurring in health and social status, particularly of women and children.

'If we continue to ignore the women's situation can we ever hope to attain Health for All, even long after the year 2000.'
– Dr Halfdan Mahler, 1985.

# Appendix 4

Details of my mother's book:

*Stover, The Story of a School*
ISBN 0 907854 01 X
Copyright Stover School 1984


and of Great-aunt Jessie's book:

*Jessie's Journey*
*Triumph and Tragedy in the Andes*
Edited by Jenny Coombe
With a foreword by Nigel Nicholson

ISBN 0 907956 025
Published
by New Forest Leaves
Burley
Ringwood, Hampshire
BH24 4BA


Note also:

*Jewels of Cambodia*
By Brenda Sloggett,
which has an interesting introduction to this country
ISBN 1 – 85078 – 637 –2
www.authenticmedia.co.uk